Mistress Ruby Ties It Together

Robin Shamburg

MISTRESS RUBY TIES IT TOGETHER

A Dominatrix Takes On Sex, Power,

and the Secret Lives of Upstanding Citizens

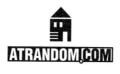

ATRANDOM.COM

NEW YORK

ATRANDOM and colophon are registered trademarks of Random House, Inc.

Library of Congress Cataloging-in-Publication Data
Shamburg, Robin.
Mistress Ruby ties it together: a dominatrix takes on sex, power, and the secret lives of upstanding citizens / Robin Shamburg.
p. cm.
ISBN 0-8129-9154-0
1. Sexual dominance and submission—New York (State)—New York—Case studies. 2. Sadomasochism—New York (State)—New York—Case studies. I. Title.
HQ79.S527 2001
306.77'5'09747—dc21   00-066481

Random House website: www.atrandom.com

Manufactured in the United States on acid-free paper

2 4 6 8 9 7 5 3

First Edition

FOR MY GRANDMOTHER

Contents

PART III

THE COOLDOWN

Mistress Ruby Ties It Together

Introduction

Several years ago, somewhere between college graduation and the commencement of responsible adulthood, I took a job at an S&M parlor in midtown Manhattan. It was there that I became Mistress Ruby, confessor-for-hire. I diapered doctors, judged judges, and bore witness to the lusts, fantasies, and fears of some of the city's most powerful businessmen. Eventually, I began writing for a newspaper called *New York Press,* where I chronicled these adventures in my weekly column, "Mistress Ruby's Whipping Post."

For the next two years, my dual identities—dominatrix and columnist—would enhance and inspire each other, and occasionally even compete in their struggle for—pardon the expression—dominance. Thanks to both careers, and the opportunities they've created, I'm proud to say that responsible adulthood hasn't caught up with me just yet.

It was never my plan to become a dominatrix, not for writing grist, nor in the name of Experience. I came to this career the way most people come to theirs—just part of the dubious dance between intention and accident, with a dash of quick-fix necessity cutting in. In the early 1990s, my best friend, Desi, and I had a job shooting karaoke videos for the Asian market—that is, music videos that play behind the drunken performers in the karaoke bars of Kuala Lumpur, Tokyo, and Bangkok.

Our budget was so meager that I was required not only to produce and paint scenery, but to star in these three-minute features as well. It seemed I had a real knack for portraying the boyfriend-stealing vixen; in a constant state of icy hauteur, my signature gesture was to toss my drink into the cheating lover's face. Who could know that these special talents would foretell my career in paid domination?

At some point in our travels, Desi and I met a young filmmaker who was funding her first feature by working as a professional dominatrix. This we found intriguing—it sounded much more innovative than shaking down relatives or maxing out your credit cards. We'd lived in the city all our lives; we thought we had a pretty good idea of what the job entailed. And we'd seen plenty of filmmakers sell their souls for celluloid fame; that someone might sell her body, if she had one worth selling, seemed like just another part of the auteur work ethic.

So we were surprised when she told us that, in fact, her job did not involve sex, nor was it illegal in the great state of New York. But we were absolutely staggered when we found out that she'd actually managed to raise the money she needed, and was meeting the substantial postproduction costs by selling off the rest of her fetish wardrobe.

Money? No sex? Cool clothes? This, we felt, was worth looking into.

A few story leads later, I found myself in the mistress lounge of one of Manhattan's premier S&M parlors. I'd been visiting the place, on and off, for almost a month, interviewing the dominatrices, sitting in on sessions, and mastering the two most important mistressing skills: watching television and ordering food for delivery. By then I'd decided that I would write about what I'd been witnessing. An article, a script—I didn't know exactly what it would be, but I did know that this world fired my imagination like nothing I'd ever seen before.

Eventually, the inevitable happened. One of the mistresses suggested that I try my hand at a session—purely for the sake of journalistic accuracy, of course. I shied and shuffled like a virgin bride, but finally I figured, what the hell? Jane Goodall didn't study primates by sitting at home watching PBS. Why shouldn't I do a little fieldwork? My new friends assured me I'd be a natural, that I already possessed the two main prerequisites for the job: must be a "people person"; must look beautiful when angry.

And so, amid much giggling and whispered asides, they helped me prepare for my first client, a dungeon regular whose session, they told me, would be simple and fun, the perfect maiden voyage. Once I was dressed, made up, pep-talked, and pointed in the direction of Dungeon #1, they informed me that I would also need a "mistress name"—my *nom de whip,* if you will. They surveyed me from every angle. "You look like a Ruby," Mistress Craven pronounced. The other girls nodded vigorously. Once I figured out that they weren't calling me a *rube,* it sounded like a nice-enough name—different but not too weird, with the same initial in case, I guess, I happened to own anything monogrammed. Then it was showtime.

The fattest guy I'd ever seen shirtless stood before me in Dungeon #1. We stared at each other for a long time—me, a nervous freshman in leather mufti; him, an investment banker encased in three hundred pounds of excess flesh. Finally he spoke: "I have a Christ complex," he said. "I want to die for you." His session, as he explained it, was for me to hang him from the St. Andrew's cross— a set of wooden beams built into the wall—through an elaborate pulley system of ropes, metal hooks, and, as far as I could tell, a blatant disregard for Newtonian physics. "Then, as I am dying, I would like you to take these pushpins"—he produced a pocketful of multicolored tacks—"and pierce my feet with them." He gently took my left foot into his palm and demonstrated—with his fingers—the proper pressure points for pushpin pushing.

I shuddered slightly and told him that while I never draw blood on the first date, as a good Catholic, I would be more than happy to re-create the Passion of Christ with him. So we spent the next fifty minutes improvising, with him as the dying Son of God. I took all the other parts—Mary Magdalene, Pontius Pilate, Joseph of Arimathea, and so forth. We even took a little detour to the Garden of Gethsemane so that I could make like an Apostle and abandon him for a quick bathroom break.

It was the strangest hour I'd ever spent with another human being—intensely intimate, absolutely comical; there were points when I felt like I was getting paid just to keep a straight face. And yet here was this complete stranger, a guy right off the street, revealing to me his most deeply held secrets, his failings and lapses of faith—all of which we acted out through our little Easter pageant. When I rolled the "stone" (a leather footstool) away from his "tomb" (a six-by-six metal cage) and pronounced him "risen," he broke down and wept at the catharsis of it all.

Besides being $150 richer, I actually felt like I'd done something, I don't know, benevolent. My new coworkers, however, had not been quite so charitable. I later found out that throwing the new girl to a difficult or especially bizarre client was a kind of mistress hazing ritual, intended to weed out the faint of heart. But I'd survived it, and I'd found my calling. My life as Mistress Ruby had officially begun.

So I spent the next two years, off and on, working as a dominatrix to subsidize my writing habit. In time, I sent some of my dungeon stories to the editors at *New York Press,* who began publishing my notes from the S&M underground. Like my fellow mistresses, I'd been enjoying the traditional double life—slacker/leather goddess—but with the column I'd gained a third identity. What can I say? I've always been an overachiever.

I've never had any big predilection for pain or sexual perversion. I tend to think there's a reason they call it a *spice*—a little goes a long way. My time in the dungeon has done nothing to change this opinion. What I did bring to mistressing, however, was my endless fascination with people and their stories—the more secret and unsavory the better. In the end, I think that's what most dungeon clients are really looking for—not so much a whipping arm but a listening ear, someone to bear witness to their inner lives.

When I first came to the dungeon, I was a rube; when I came out, however, everybody else was an expert. It seemed like the pop explosion of S&M had spared no one. When you can walk into any mall and purchase some kind of studded leather doodad, when S&M

is used to sell everything from candy bars to gym memberships, it's pretty safe to say that *fetish* has entered the national lexicon. In fact you can look it up; it's in the dictionary, in its S&M context, right between, appropriately enough, *fetid* and *fetlock.*

Unfortunately, all this mainstreaming has spread a deceptive sort of knowledge about the scene, a misinformation as potentially hazardous as swabbing a freshly welted ass with a tube of Ben-Gay. Suddenly, you don't have to have been there to be an authority. But faithful viewing of HBO's *Real Sex* won't unlock the mysteries of S&M any more than *National Geographic Explorer* will teach you how to scale the Matterhorn. All it's done is smarten up the puns, the punch lines, and—here's the hazardous part—provided us with a battery of pat, cocktail-party answers about what are really very complex matters of human behavior.

I am not at all interested in contributing to this phenomenon. So when it came time to write this book, I developed a couple of criteria. First, unlike the experts, I would not speak for the clients I've seen as if they were one single-willed, perversion-seeking organism: *These guys, you see, they have so much power at work—at the end of the day they need somebody else to tell them what to do!* Each had his own history, passion, and heartache, and a special way of getting under my skin or making my day, or both. I've tried to relay these moments as faithfully as possible, subject as they are to my own perceptions and fantasies—whatever was going on in my life at the time.

My other guideline was that if you can see it on cable TV, you won't see it here. There will be no cross-dressers or foot fetishists in these pages; in fact, the only person who ends up dressing like a dog is me, and that was not for sexual gratification, that was for my grandmother.

Instead, I've cut to all the good parts, the exceptions and the outtakes and the occasional flashes of clarity. The personal dramas. In the world of commercialized perversion, these moments of realness are what made the experience remarkable. I hope that they are an adventure for you as well.

PART I

THE SESSIONS

STILL LIFE WITH JAILBAIT

What can I tell you about the man we used to call Chester the Molester?

Chester and I began our little tango during my early days at Lady Leona's Reformatory. It was my second week on the job, and it was also Yom Kippur. I mention this because I'd just learned a little-known fact about world religions: a vast number of dungeon clients are Jewish, and they don't often elect to atone in an S&M parlor.

So, business was *dreck*. Worse, my unemployment checks were running out and I was seriously beginning to reconsider my career choice. Then, one fateful afternoon, Ida, the phone lady, called me into the office, quickly and surreptitiously, so as not to alert my coworkers. This, I'd learned, was a sign that good things were afoot.

She locked the door behind me. "David called," she said. "He wants to meet you."

"Diaper David? Or David, throw-eggs-at-me David?"

"*David* David. *Leona's* David."

"Whoa," I said. If she had told me that *Michelangelo's* David wanted to spend the afternoon with me, I wouldn't have been more tickled. For although we called him Chester the Molester, Leona, our boss, called him her business partner.

Which he was, if you consider recruiting jailbait to satisfy his sugar-daddy cravings to be a sound example of fiscal planning. He was a real VIP to us Reformatory girls, never took appointments in the actual dungeon, but at Leona's apartment, this tacky, overly mirrored high-rise for shady international types (you could pay rent in cash) and the nouveau riche, which Chester bankrolled.

"He'll be picking you up in a half-hour. You want I should steam your Catholic school uniform?"

I shook my head. "Too obvious. When I was seventeen, no one even wore their school uniforms to school. I've got something much better."

"Is it slutty enough for the creep?"

"If you're underage, it is."

"That sick SOB," muttered Ida, who had a school-age daughter. "Better bring the uniform anyway."

This was Chester's trip: spending time with a girl who was either jailbait or mighty convincing as such; introducing this girl to the ways of sick and twisted middle-aged rich guys; corrupting this girl; and paying handsomely for the privilege.

Now, I was closer to twenty-five than to twenty, already well corrupted and with a flair for the dramatic—not to mention a serious financial deficit. And while I'm not naive enough to presume that I single-handedly saved the schoolgirls of America from Chester's gross advances, I still believe that seeing me was a far more appropriate outlet for his disgusting desires.

Besides, if you think about it, the role didn't really require me to *do* anything. In fact, the whole point was to do nothing: *don't* talk about where I was when Richard Nixon resigned (kindergarten); *don't* mention my familiarity with the entire *Ass Masters* oeuvre; and so forth.

So Chester picked me up and whisked me off to Lady Leona's lair. We rode in utter silence, each stealing little appraising glances at the other, like some kind of weird first date, a girl and her uncle.

In fact, Chester did bear a stunning resemblance to my uncle Sal—
disconcerting, to say the least, and something I sensed would loom
much larger in the hours to come.

The only thing that broke the silence was when we stopped at a
light and a gaggle of obviously gay boys swirled around the car.
Chester turned to me, real confidential-like. "Ya know, I useta suck
a mean cock," he said, "before there was all that AIDS."

I nodded solemnly and swallowed, hard. I figured that was what
an eighteen-year-old would do. I spent the rest of the ride trying to
get in touch with my inner Lolita, that part of me that was unspoiled
but oh-so-ripe for corruption. This was to be my schtick, my persona: a sweet but secretly tartish teen, fresh out of an all-girls
Catholic high school, the kind of institution that guys like Chester
can only fantasize about.

So Chester and I are lounging around Leona's apartment, which
has that painful immigrant "we've-finally-made-it-in-America"
decor, all leather, mirrors, and beveled glass surfaces. He's sitting on
the sectional leather sofa wearing a pair of queen-size pantyhose
and nothing else; I've been talked into the old school uniform, complete with kneesocks and clip-on plaid tie.

Ron Jeremy sucks his own dick on the big-screen TV as I sit at
this IKEA minidesk, pretending to be in class. Meanwhile Chester,
balled up like a waterbug—and only slightly more attractive than
Mr. Jeremy—attempts to fellate himself as well. The doppelganger
image is overwhelming. I am wedged between two bookends of a
hairy, fleshy hell.

Chester rolls himself back into an upright position.

"Let's pretend I am your teacher," he says, "and I have switched
today's instructional film with this—" He waves his jack-off hand at
the screen. "And now you're sitting in class and watching it. What
do you do?"

I think about it—what I'd really do, and what would be the most
titillating thing to tell Chester the Molester.

"I'd—I'd maybe masturbate . . . ?"

"Yess . . . yesss. Very good, yesss. And what else?"

"I'd, uh, like, show all the other girls how to masturbate . . . ?"

"And how would you show them that?" Chester asks, clearly inspired.

Shit, I think. Now I've gone too far. I've talked myself into a corner and am expected to diddle my way out of it. No can do—you never pull out the big guns on your first encounter, if ever. Too bad for him I'm not really eighteen.

"Like, I'd call you back into class and have you give us all, like, a lesson . . . ?"

Suffice it to say that Mistress Ruby went to the head of the class with that answer. The mental image of himself masturbating before a classroom of plaid-skirted geometry students while Ron Jeremy drinks his own ejaculate in the background was plenty enough to send my friend over the edge. Chester soiled his nice fresh pair of queen-size pantyhose and pledged his undying sugar-daddiness to me. Then he drove me back to the dungeon.

How did it all turn out, you ask? Well, this was merely the beginning of a long and lovely friendship, in which Mistress Ruby and Chester, Child Molester, rent pornies, call phone sex, pee in the tub, and do pretty much every juvenile thing short of setting our farts on fire. I ended up seeing him, sometimes often, sometimes seldom, for years after that. My world and welcome to it.

SISTER RUBY, MISTRESS SUPERIOR

What's amazing to me is how you can see the same client for weeks, sometimes even months, and yet remain completely ignorant of his raison d'etre, his real session. Chances are he's oblivious to it too. But he'll keep coming back, whether out of faith, fear, or spousal familiarity—*yeah, my mistress beats me like an old shoe*—until one day the session clicks; the meaning becomes magically, terribly clear. Then you've got to decide if it's something you want to deal with.

Joseph was a client I'd been seeing on-again, off-again for nearly four months—a respectable run in this business. Joseph himself was a bit of an anachronism. He resembled a young Al Pacino and dressed like an extra from *The Rockford Files*—checkered sports coat, wide of lapel and heavy on the topstitching—and smoked a brand of cigarettes (Kents, I believe—great flavor, low "tar") that they stopped making during the Carter administration. Kind of unscrupulous, but not quite a bad guy—the used-car salesman caught up in some shady doings; eventually he helps Jim Rockford bring down the *real* villains.

Anyway, every so often—twice a month, once a month, every other day for a fortnight—Joseph would walk his seventies self into my dungeon. Don't ask me what precipitated his visits—troubles at home? fat residuals check?—it's anybody's guess. Our sessions could at best be described as lackluster: He'd rub my feet; I'd bark a few basic insults.

Then I'd lock him in the cage to do his business into some tissues, leave the room to order myself some dinner or to chat with more compelling characters—the delivery boy from Habib's Falafel, our meter reader, and so on.

But time after time, Joseph kept showing up, a continuing source of puzzlement to me. I was never actually convinced that he enjoyed this treatment—there was something too expectant about him as he stared up from my shoes. Something that, when I detected it, made me feel obliged to stifle that yawn. Because really, it wasn't Joseph's job to entertain me, I told myself. Besides, he tipped very well and kept coming back, a pretty reliable sign of customer satisfaction. Free country, right?

And then one evening, full of piss and vinegar (and, admittedly, three hundred dollars richer than I had planned) I decided to stage my own dungeon version of civil disobedience. Instead of perching atop the punishment horse and proffering Joseph my boot, I sat smack down on the floor across from him and stared him down. I had decided earlier, when he'd booked his appointment, that I didn't care if he never saw me again; I figured I could make him do something if only through my refusal to do *anything*.

I thought wrong. Joseph just sat and stared back blankly like some bad blind date, as if waiting for us to magically end up in bed together. Maybe he thought we were participating in a John Cage performance piece; some kind of experimental boredom-torture.

Either way, my little sit-down strike was backfiring on me. It was time to enforce Plan B. This had to do with me dashing out to the transvestite closet and raping it of its most luridly slutty garments, then forcing Joseph, at whip-point, to don that slut gear and parade about like the featured dancer at Bob's Klassy Lady. I'd recently discovered that a little impromptu cross-dressing can work wonders on difficult clients.

But the force was not with me that evening; some other mistress had already picked the closet clean. All that remained was this ripped, Queen Elizabeth–style gown in a fabric that looked like upholstery and a few mismatched, size-12 pumps, the heels hobbled to nubs. That, and my old Catholic-school-uniform sweater—iron-on emblem and all—which I had given up for stolen weeks ago.

I threw the sweater over my shoulders and grabbed a mini slide rule that one of my more studious coworkers had left sitting on top of the television.

I walked back into the dungeon with renewed purpose. Joseph was still sitting on the floor. "Joseph, you have won the distinction of being the most boring slave I have ever seen. Consider this your prize." I handed him the slide rule.

"Now. If you do not utilize your award in some manner entertaining to me, you can drag your Sansabelt-slacked ass out of here and never return."

He stared back at me, clearly confused. "But I haven't used one of these since high school, Mistress Ruby. What exactly do you want me to do with it?"

"I don't care if you stick it up your rectum, Joseph," I replied.

He seemed to genuinely consider the suggestion; still, he offered no response. Joseph 1, Mistress Ruby 0.

Now I was infuriated.

"I mean that you are so boring that you do not merit my cruel ministrations, so I am forced to request that you do violence to yourself." Still no reply.

"I said strike thyself, dullard!"

Joseph began slapping himself across his palm with the plastic slide rule, tentatively at first, then gaining momentum as I egged him on: "Faster! Harder! Let's hear those cries of agony! Now switch hands! I wanna see some welts! On the knuckles! Harder! I can't *hear* you!" And so on.

Joseph, much to his credit, kept the pace like a pro. To his discredit, he stared at my chest the whole time. After he was done, I asked him about it.

"You know better than to look at me, Joseph. What was that all about?"

He cast his eyes humbly downward. "Actually, Mistress, I was noticing the emblem on your sweater—would you mind telling me where it's from?"

Okay, it was time to ease up—but just a little. I pulled off the sweater. "Saints Peter and Paul," I said, holding the patch up to the dim dungeon light. "You know, you rob one to pay the other. It's where I went to grammar school. And where I learned the ruler trick," I added, perhaps unnecessarily.

"And what's that hat Paul is wearing?" he asked.

"Tahini sauce, I believe."

Joseph fell silent for a long few moments—probably gathering the courage for his next request. Oh, but I could just smell it coming. "And do you have, you know, the rest of the outfit?"

Oh, Christ, I thought—*just when I thought things were starting to go well, he's got to trot* this *one out.*

"Yes, Joseph," I replied wearily, "I do indeed have it all—the teeny-weeny ankle socks, the regulation blouse with the Peter Pan collar, the plaid vest and plaid skirt with which I will tantalize you into remembering those naughty schoolboy days, in which you yanked my braids and I, the naughty school*girl,* kicked your ass from one end of the school yard to the other.

"Or perhaps you were older, and stalked me home from school in your car, until the day I stepped up to the driver's-side window of your late-model sedan and slapped you repeatedly across your evil, greasy, stalker's face as you sat with your stained, ugly pervert's trousers around your ankles. Yes, I have it, I have it, *I have it!*"

"Actually, I meant the *other* uniform," he stammered. "You know—the habit, the wimple. The support hose with the runs in them?"

"The close-cropped hair and the arthritic fingers with the Rosary entwined between?" I asked. "The heaving shelf of a bosom, the vague scent of Ivory Soap, chicken soup, and urine? The indignation, repression, and wrath born of sexual frustration and years of thankless servitude to a corrupt and misogynist institution?" "Yes." He nodded. "Yes, yes, yes!" And then Joseph smiled the smile of a man who was finally understood; a man whose fantasy was on the menu.

"So now I'm a nun," I said. "And then what do we do? Are you a priest straying from his vows, maybe? Another nun? My lesbian-nun lover?"

"No, nothing *weird* like that," he scoffed. "I just want, you know, for you to catch me, like, playing with myself in the cloakroom or something."

Jesus with a strap-on, I thought. "You mean you've wasted all these sessions boring the hell out of me when all you wanted was for me to dress up funny and catch you jerking off? Why didn't you say something and spare me the mind-numbing tedium?"

"I figured you're a pro, you would know," Joseph replied.

I seized the slide rule and rapped him a good one. "Well, it looks like Mr. Joseph has made a little rhyme—hasn't he? Mr. Joseph is a poet and he doesn't even know it. Does he, class?" Like a magic wand, I waved my ruler across a row of paddles. Suddenly they became a room full of terrified seventh-graders.

"Now march your ass into that corner and don't let me see your hands straying anywhere that our Lord wouldn't want them to."

So Joseph did march, impure thoughts spawning and humping (missionary position, of course) in his head. And lo—his hands did stray, and Sister Ruby did rain the wrath of God down upon him.

I'd like to tell you more of what happened, but patience, perseverance, boys and girls. You'll just have to wait until next time, when Mr. Joseph is reminded that small things amuse small minds and a guilty conscience needs no accuser. Meanwhile, eyes forward, heads up, and cut the dialogue, people—what, were you all vaccinated with a phonograph needle?

FANTASY THEORY 101

Not long after my standoff with Joseph, I became interested in finding a reliable way to identify and carry out the true wishes of any given client—a Rosetta stone for fantasy, if you will. Of course, I never completely cracked the code, but I did develop the following guidelines:

The Proclaimed Fantasy

This is what a man presents to the world as his most heartfelt desire. It rarely has anything to do with what actually arouses him; it has everything to do with how he'd like to be perceived. You'll notice that it sounds very much like a Personals ad: *I would like a girl who's outgoing and fun, who has a nice smile. It doesn't matter what she looks like, as long as she's sincere.*

The Locker-Room Fantasy

This is what a man will tell his guy friends in those charming male moments of bonding. It may or may not involve alcohol and belching competitions. Like the Proclaimed Fantasy, it has everything to do with how he'd like to be perceived. But since it's a strictly guy-to-guy disclosure, its larger purpose is to emphasize that he is definitely, absolutely not a homosexual. *Christ, but wouldn't you just love to fuck that girl with the tits from Accounting? Maybe some night we can tag-team her!*

The Fantasy Fit for a Dominatrix

This is what a man will feel free to disclose in a paying situation. Safe in the knowledge that you are a Professional Pervert, and have probably seen much worse, he feels free to let it all hang out. If that doesn't liberate him, at least he can remind himself that while he may occasionally want to bark like a dog, you, freak lady, are sexually deviant all day long! It goes: *I would like you to dress like a cheerleader and slap me around, maybe gag me with your bra. It doesn't matter what else you do, as long as I can see your tits through your sweater.*

The Final Analysis

This is the fantasy that is never spoken aloud. In fact, the guy may not even realize it as his ultimate sexual dream. It is up to you, the seasoned dominatrix, to listen closely as he recites his dominatrix-safe fantasy. Apply the twin presses of perception and compassion, and what you will extract is that rare and beautiful liquid, the essential oil of fantasy: *I would like you to dress* me *as a cheerleader. A slutty cheerleader, the walking cock-holster of the entire football team. It doesn't matter what you, my lesbian lover, do to me, as long as you remember that I love to be sodomized. Oh, and by the way, I have these really big tits.*

ENEMAS: A FAIRY TALE

Craven and Destina were two Puerto Rican goth girls and the senior doms at Lady Leona's Reformatory. To me, Craven and Destina served as a living reminder that certain kinds of people will continuously reappear in your life. I'd met these two before; they were the pajama-party power brokers, the girls who decided who sat next to whom and who got her slumbering hand draped into a mug of urine.

For a while, their chosen playmate was young Helene, whom they had picked up one chilly autumn afternoon while shoplifting at Macy's. As the legend goes, they found the girl clinging to a rack of parkas in the outerwear department, dropped to her knees, sobbing uncontrollably.

One can only imagine what they must have looked like to Helene, looming over her in their cheap, St. Mark's Place Satan-wear. Whatever it was, she stopped crying. "It was like she was *expecting* us, no lie," Destina was fond of reminiscing.

To me, Craven and Destina were like a set of sinister Christmas ornaments—two scheming elves wearing too much eyeliner. To Helene, however, they were no less than a heavenly apparition to the faithful. She rose to her feet, wiped her nose on a Gore-Tex sleeve, and began following them without a word. It was her very first day in the States.

Helene had fled from one of those Eastern bloc countries so obscure that every time I tried to picture it, the image came out grainy and sepia-tinted. The kind of place where consumerism was a revolutionary concept, where newly erected billboards instructed *This Is Where Merchants May Advertise Their Products.* On the third floor of Macy's Herald Square, Helene had been physically overwhelmed by the wealth of available goods here, and so she sobbed and hugged their bounty.

Later on, when she got the language together, she explained to us that days before her brave journey, she had consulted with the wise woman of her town. This woman, whose specialties were spell casting and the vanquishing of "demons unique to the unwed virgin"— abortions, we figured—had, since the advent of capitalism, turned a pretty profit foretelling futures in this uncertain age. She told Helene that she should dare to defy her family and head for the United States. "You will ride American decadence to stardom beyond imagination," she had prophesied, dropping Helene's coins neatly in the slot between her foam falsies and her mastectomy scar.

In the States, the woman continued, Helene would meet an individual who would teach her what she needed to know to launch her magnificent future. Among that rack of parkas, she knew she had found that person, for she—quite perceptively, I thought—recognized Craven and Destina as a single unit. Once, I even caught Helene gazing lovingly over a copy of *The Seven Habits of Highly Effective People,* framing the dominatrices with misty eyes. "Svengali," she whispered; I would almost swear to it.

If Craven and Destina were her star-sent instructresses, then Macy's Herald Square had proven to be a first-rate classroom. It was there that Helene received a crash course in the finer points of supply-side economics: how to spot a surveillance camera at twenty paces, how to distract the dressing-room attendant while your compatriots shove merchandise down their pants, how to stroll past the security guards with just the right measure of youthful high spirits and nonchalance.

Snatching a cab from a flock of nurses, they whisked her off to the dungeon. Unbeknown to the two dominatrices, they had just taught young Helene the most valuable lesson of all: that as far as goods and services went, Helene would never wait on line again.

No one recognized the full value of the day's take better than Leona, our scheming pimp of a boss. She, too, had come to the States with a singular ambition—in her case, to become a great, rich lady. To that end, she had taken the name of her idol, a certain New York hotelier and another famous female boss. Unfortunately, in the process, she'd adopted many of her managerial strategies as well.

So if Helene's vernacular had a word for *tricky, insincere cunt,* that would surely have been the word that came to mind when she first met Leona. Oh, the tears that were shed, the homecoming of hugs as our employer opened her hearth to this wretched refuse, this friendless orphan, her fellow immigrant. By all accounts, if there had been a fatted calf grazing on the premises, Leona probably would have killed it.

Ida, the phone lady, witnessed the touching scene. "You could just see the rubles," she reported, "multiplying in the old clam's head." Needless to say, Ida was a woman whose paycheck was not big enough to cover anyone's bullshit.

But why was Lady Leona so eager to lift her light beside our dungeon door? Because even in Helene's tear-stained, tempest-tost state, the girl was exquisitely, undeniably beautiful. And by beautiful, I don't mean supermodel; I mean *supernatural,* as though she had wafted to earth from another world.

In a way, this was true. She'd reached adulthood unsullied by American influence; she'd never downloaded or StairMastered or microwaved; she'd never claimed to be having a Big Mac Attack or a Bad Hair Day. And, by God, you could see it on her—an untouched, rarefied perfection.

Women didn't even think of envying her—you would just as

soon be jealous of, say, a newborn baby, or a Fabergé egg. Nor did men try to possess her; it would be like expecting to marry an apparition. Hers was a virginity that went beyond simple chastity, something that compelled our clients to worship and stare, to beg to bask in her grace. A privilege, Leona realized, for which they'd pay handsomely.

If Helene was taken aback by the force of her welcome or by the eccentricities of her new surroundings—the Kleenex boxes bursting with condoms, the auto-da-fé decor—she took it all in stride. Plausible, too, seemed the terms of her new employment—that is, reminding wealthy men what it was like to sing for their suppers.

"We are a private crusade to reform the bourgeoisie," Leona told her, communicating in a crude pidgin dialect of gestures and grade-school French. The rest of us, loath to lose our jobs, scrambled around to outfit our stunning new recruit in the plastic teddies and the spiked brassieres that were the uniform of our movement.

Tabula rasa, Helene went along with all of it. After all, what did she have to lose? The role asked almost nothing of her. Her one official duty was to help Leona free our clients from the shackles of capitalism. Unofficially, she was required to help Craven and Destina chop up their boundless supply of cheap cocaine (which they liked to do on Leona's copy of *Walking with Jesus*). As long as she made sure that her ever-expanding nest of shoplifted clothes—which doubled as her bed—didn't block the heating ducts, she was welcome to set up housekeeping at Lady Leona's Reformatory.

But Leona was no fool; she recognized that the golden goose had come to roost in her dungeon. And she was very superstitious—she believed that one-breasted soothsayer's prophecy. It was not difficult to see how quickly a beauty of Helene's caliber could be "discovered" on the streets of New York City, transformed into a model or a VJ or a soap opera star—and plucked from Leona's pocket forever.

Legal alien to illegal alien, she took the girl aside and advised her to do her shoplifting only between 9:00 and 10:00 a.m., taking a cab both ways, and always with a chaperone. Also, she felt it was important that Helene understand her rights.

"Immigration Patrol can't ask for your green card until 10:01," she told the wide-eyed Helene. "And don't let them deport you before lunchtime. By law, they're supposed to give you a sandwich first."

So that was how Leona's favorite employee became the dungeon's most pampered prisoner, locked in the hole twenty-three hours a day. What she couldn't steal, we loaned her (and had stolen from us). What she couldn't get delivered, we fetched for her. What she didn't know, she learned through cable TV: that evil twins exist (*All My Children*); that an estranged husband is your deadliest foe (Lifetime: Television for Women); and that the best way to settle an argument is to brain your opponent with a folding metal chair (the WWF).

But even within the relative security of the dungeon, we were required to hide her, and hide things from her—namely, certain clients. Leona didn't want her having contact with any men—from entertainment guys to the overly amorous—that might start to get ideas about Helene's future.

In the end, however, Leona's paranoia was no match for the soothsayer's prediction. American decadence, a mysterious benefactor; Helene's destiny was immutable. Unfortunately, the prophecy failed to mention this benefactor's passion for recreational bowel cleansing. And that's how Enema Pete, one of our wealthiest regulars, managed to slip through the cracks and into Helene's life. Providing us, along the way, with a battery of loathsome puns that I'm sure you can imagine for yourself.

We don't know exactly how they managed to meet, but we think it was the result of poor communication among staff members. Leona wasn't around that week and so none of us were sure of his security-risk rating—this fluctuated along with Leona's paranoia—and so the protocol was unclear. To be on the safe side—and to ensure more money for ourselves—we simply told Helene to hide.

The trouble was, with most forbidden clients, Helene's usual hiding place was in the bathroom, behind the shower curtain. She had no way of knowing—and someone neglected to tell her—that this was the absolute worst place to conceal herself from Enema Pete.

So that's probably where their eyes first met—not, as the song goes, across a crowded room, but in one very cramped bathroom as Pete liberated three Fleet enemas into the dungeon toilet bowl.

Maybe he wasn't the one she eloped with. But all the evidence seems to point in his direction. One, we never saw him after that; two, both Helene and her cache of shoplifted gains were gone the very next morning. When Ida reported to work, she found a wide-open window, and a crate of Fleet enemas was missing from the supply cabinet.

But she wouldn't have known to check there if not for the final piece of evidence, which we found at the bottom of the fire escape: no glass slipper, clear and precious, but a crumpled plastic enema bottle, which had clearly been used for its intended purpose.

Which leaves us to wonder: Did Helene and Pete, in their romantic fervor, stop for a "quickie" in the dungeon alley? Was this meant as some kind of slap in the face to us, her S&M stepsisters? Could the bottle be nothing more than a false clue, something meant to throw us off the real story? Or maybe we were just supposed to take comfort, even inspiration, in the notion that there was an enema prince out there for all of us, that sometimes, in the midst of decadence and corruption, fairy tales can still come true.

BELOW THE BELT

It's pretty safe to say that most men have no desire, latent or otherwise, to get kicked in the balls. Me, I've met a couple too many guys who've enjoyed this, viciously and repeatedly, to chalk it up to coincidence. It's the kind of session where I find myself double- and triple-checking the request. First, I want to make sure my hearing hasn't failed me. Then I need to know that this client is in full possession of his faculties, a consenting adult with no apparent psychological problems—beyond the obvious.

Finally, we've both got to agree that I won't be held responsible for any fertility problems that might someday arise. Once we've defined our terms—and I can shake the image of a petri dish teeming with shattered spermatozoa—I'll proceed with my usual vigor. I promise you that.

But it's a scene I'll never fully understand. I don't know about you, but all my life I've been told that you just don't do that, some things are sacred, lay off the family jewels. At least, that's the male opinion. And groin vulnerability seems to create a kind of absolute

brotherhood among men, an empathy that transcends all other be-
liefs, even logic itself.

For example, one night a friend and I were discussing Hitler and
his purported single testicle. We were trying to figure out how, exactly, he'd lost it, but no luck (this was long before the Internet).

"Ooh, but that's gotta be rough," my friend concluded, cupping
his crotch in sympathy. I understand that he was speaking for all
men, not just the Führer; still, you can't ignore the implication: *Poor
Hitler!*

But if, among men, groin pain can inspire compassion, however
secondhand, for even the most unworthy, consider the reaction of
the fairer sex. For us, nothing says "laff riot" quite like the sight of
a man crumpling to the ground in the throes of scrotal agony.
Doesn't matter who it is. It could be Jesus Christ, or Santa Claus,
and we'd still feel glee, even a touch of pride. A good swift groin
shot represents the female's ability to survive in an increasingly
hostile world—it's a guaranteed victory, kind of like a get-out-of-
rape-free card.

Somewhere between these two extremes, there's got to be a mid-
point of reason. Personally, I believe that if anyone larger and
stronger than me—and let's face it, to the average-sized woman,
that's the average-sized man—approaches me with the intent to do
violence, he's already hitting below the belt. Anything I've got to do
to gain advantage—bite, pull hair, or run like a rabbit—seems like a
perfectly fair strategy. If you've ever had the pleasure of witnessing
a real bar brawl, you'll see that most men secretly share this opinion;
I've yet to see a man unwilling to fight like a girl if it means saving
his own ass.

But I'm not talking reason here; I'm talking S&M. In the dungeon, I'm fighting for my livelihood, not my life, and so my personal views on self-defense don't matter one bit. And as a
dominatrix, what compels a man to enjoy this particular sensation
is not my primary concern. In order to play my part, I've got to
think of pain as pain, none more taboo than another. In other words,

I'll provide the trappings and ritual; don't expect any extra sympathy just because it happens to be happening to your yams, tough guy.

More so than most scenes, nut kicking is an extremely stylized event. I've performed the session more than a dozen times with the same three aficionados, and if I'd put in the exact same performance every time, they would have all limped home satisfied. At its core, a groin-kicking session is literally a battle of the sexes. To give it the necessary bite, I've got to take the extreme girlie position.

Here's how it works in a session. Me and Dick Leakey are standing around somewhere—could be an art museum, could be a 7-Eleven. He is meek and unassuming, but twitchy. He strikes up a conversation with me, something innocuous. But then he lets slip some unsavory comment: "Venus de Milo's got nothin' on you, Cupcake—you got yourself some *legs.*"

Then Mr. Leakey tries to touch me in an inappropriate manner, usually around the waist or shoulders. This is my cue to wriggle free, step back one and a half paces in six-inch stilettos, spin around one whole turn, throw my head back and growl—picture James Brown minus the duckwalk—and karate kick him in the scrotum with cruel dispatch.

I then proceed to dismantle my would-be attacker. Once he's prone, I deliver a few more perfunctory blows to his crotch until he begs to be spared. Finally, when he cries for mercy, I make the requisite speech, which goes something like this:

"While I am certain that you, a big and strong man, thought that you could harm a sweet and defenseless lady like me, I trust that we have demonstrated otherwise. For you, like all men, have a single point of vulnerability that has become my secret advantage. . . ." And so on, until Mr. Leakey is forced to admit that it was his dick that was his undoing.

There are two telling aspects to this session. The first is the dress code: short skirt, tight as a tourniquet; suntan—yes, *suntan* stockings; and high heels—a caricature of femininity. Not what I'd normally wear in a combat situation; then again, I'm not supposed to be expecting the onslaught.

But Mr. Leakey's turn-on is not about attacking me unawares. At heart, the groin-kick lover is a leg and foot enthusiast. Just as in the case of the classic fetishist, the whole of feminine sexuality is encoded in a nicely turned leg, the high arch of a shapely foot. Unlike your standard leg worshiper, however, he doesn't get his thrill from a set of passive gams.

In his case, form takes a backseat to function. He likes that female leg as an instrument of force and destruction, the leg in action. Here, the lesson learned is that a woman's leg has the power to bring not just the *man,* but his entire *manhood,* to its knees.

The second telling detail is that ending speech. It is absolutely essential to the session; it reinforces the kicking. What Mr. Leakey wants to know is that yes, his manhood is what makes him strong—the urgent demands of his throbbing member precipitated the attack; his arousal literally *gave him the balls* to proceed. But it's also what makes him weak—that which turned him on can also turn on him, swiftly and terribly. Curb your desire; beware your own genitalia. Love hurts.

These groin-kick sessions have led me to my own scrotum theory. It's about evolution; specifically, how it would seem that the Creator was sleeping at the wheel when He hung a man's testicles on the outside of the body. It's either too warm or too cold; constant adjustments must be made in order to ensure optimum fertility. And talk about vulnerable—you may as well draw a bull's-eye right below the belt buckle. Centrally located, swinging in the open, that sac is ripe for the kill. You would think that if we were merely meant to "be fruitful and multiply," God would have stashed the jewels in a safer place.

Unless we're missing the point. Maybe it wasn't some heavenly folly to handicap all that hunting, raping, and pillaging muscle mass with such delicate baggage. Maybe someone's trying to tell us that there's a little more to it than riding roughshod over the planet.

If every man shares an equal risk of certain damage, then we've got something of a standoff here. Evolution would mean developing not just brute strength, but the ability to reason and negotiate. We might have to learn that a little bit of compromise, a modicum of diplomacy, will save us a world of pain.

MARATHON MISTRESS

Hold my calls. Cancel all appointments. Double up on candy and Snapple and smokes. Wear the *sensible* stilettos. Above all, leave the wristwatch at home. I'm about to embark on a ten-hour journey with a gentleman I'll call the LPR. Together we'll explore territories both strange and familiar—long, dull stretches of flatland punctuated by steep, hardscrabble terrain. Tolls will be collected; bridges will be crossed. There will at times be a bitter struggle for control of the radio. But this is no road trip, because we've no intention of stepping outside of Dungeon #2. In terms of sheer claustrophobic intensity, "acid trip" is more like it.

An LPR—Long-Playing Regular—is a client who is known by the extraordinary duration of his session, a client who books multiple hours or days, entire weekends, sometimes even longer. Every dungeon has at least one of them. Depending on his endurance—not to mention credit rating—a single LPR might frequent several establishments the way a cagey farmer rotates his crops, careful to move to a second location before exhausting the resources of the first.

Over the course of a single session, one LPR might go through four or five mistresses, and so these clients swiftly become industry legends. There's the Hollywood producer who spent twelve hours in full-body suspension, pitching scripts as mistresses spurred him to new depths of creativity by means of a plastic flogger: *It's* Rain Man *meets* Yentl*! It's* The Deer Hunter . . . *in a supermarket!* There's the pro golfer we knew as Toodles the Terrier, who spent Christmas Day fetching a squeak toy. Or the Orthodox Jew who booked a four-hour female-transformation session on Friday afternoon, still in full makeup as sundown descended. The mistresses granted him religious asylum, and he kept the Sabbath holy in tulle and fishnets.

But whether it's with or without pain, restraints, verbal commands, or specific costuming, the LPR's session is not an S&M session in the traditional sense. I've participated enough times to recognize that it doesn't matter what we do exactly. Fact is, for most of the time, we don't seem to be doing much of anything. In that respect, a client who wants to hang upside down for fifteen hours has more in common with a guy who wants to fetch a ball for fifteen hours than a guy who wants to hang upside down for fifteen minutes. It's the marathon length of the session that's the important part—the sense of *going the distance.*

Please, come sit in on my session.

8:30 p.m.: I've never seen this LPR before, but by the time I get to him, he's already logged six hours of session. Jerry is fortyish, handsome, but with an unfortunate, prematurely soggy physique—the kind of body that says he's given up on youth, or life.

We do the standard meet-and-greet, and when asked, he expresses a mild interest in the studded paddle and bamboo cane. I position him, ass up, and give him a few sets with each, but neither seems to take. I repeat the procedure, harder this time, and again no response. It's starting to feel downright perfunctory, as if we must fulfill the minimum caning quota that session law requires. We proceed with these pleasantries for what seems like two hours, but when I allow myself a peek at the clock, it's only 9:06.

10:00 p.m.: "Given your druthers, Jerry, what would you like us to do for the next eight and a half hours?"

"I would like to do anything you would like to do, Mistress Ruby," says Jerry.

"I would like to read this August 1994 copy of *Scientific American* that I found in the supply closet, Jerry." Alas, recreational reading is not on. "Anything" does not always mean *anything* when someone is paying for it.

But Jerry does need to use the bathroom—the third time in an hour—and I see my bargaining chip. I make a deal with him: each time I let him go to the bathroom, I get to read a feature-length science article. Without interruption. Jerry trots off to the bathroom, liking this suggestion very much.

Bargaining, the constant monitoring of gifts and favors, is a popular activity with LPRs. True, this give-and-take is a staple of all session play—latex or leather? studded paddle or open palm? In the extended session, however, the things we regulate are a tad more basic—bathroom privileges, sips of water, things within a babysitter's jurisdiction.

1:00 a.m.: Two trips to the bathroom, two feature articles later, and boy does Jerry have energy! He's pinballing around the room, lighting on a chair for a second or two, popping back up, fluffing his hair in the mirror. I've let him off the proverbial leash for a good thirty minutes, just to see what he would do if left unsupervised. But now he wants me to put down my magazine and join him—hold his hand, stand at his side, check inside the supply cabinet to make sure that we're really alone. *Pay attention to me! Pay attention to me!* his manic little ballet insists.

Then he tells me he's afraid he needs to go to the bathroom again. "Jerry, you're not getting high in there, are you?" No, he protests sweatily, it's not that, not that at all. It's just that he's *afraid of* the bathroom and would like me to accompany him there. Jerry's bathroom privileges are revoked until further notice.

My anger, his denial—it's starting to feel like we're covering the Five Stages of Death. Jerry sulks and paces in the corner while I finish reading another article. It reminds me of when I was a child and my parents would leave me with the baby-sitter, how stressful those evenings were for me. I had the idea that it was my job, as the kid, to *entertain* the baby-sitter—if I didn't produce the right toys, she would think me a failure as a hostess, maybe tell the other sitters and I'd never be sat for again.

I lay this little reminiscence on Jerry, but he doesn't get the hint. I figure this means I'm with a guy who doesn't even have an eight-year-old's sense of obligation. That, or my blood sugar is plummeting fast.

1:30 a.m.: I slip out of the room to slam a few Gatorades, and notice that the dungeon is practically deserted. Only a few straggling pro doms remain. They're sympathetic to my situation, and God bless 'em—you've got to understand, I'm paying off a month's bills sitting there, bored out of my skull. Meanwhile, they're sitting on the other side of the wall, making squat. Like the real-estate agent says, location, location, location. I remind myself that 6:00 a.m. will come for everyone, no matter where anybody sits.

3:00 a.m.: Acceptance. Jerry and I have finally hit our stride. And why not? The dungeon's officially empty and it's the hour where anything goes. I notice the wedding band and wonder where his wife thinks he is.

Next thing you know, he's confessing to me like I'm the bartender in a Sinatra song. Seems that the selfish but not-quite-evil dame left him nearly a month ago. Now he can't seem to help himself; he's spent the last few weeks divesting himself of his old life before it all gets drawn into lots by the lawyers. In the middle of his unburdening, he helps himself to a sip of my Gatorade. By dungeon law, this is an audacious and eminently punishable offense. I let it slide, but allow myself a peek at the clock.

5:05 a.m.: Apropos of nothing, we start talking about the space program. I'd read only hours before that if we wanted to put a man on the moon again, it would take NASA a full ten years before we had the technology together to do it. "We're rusty, spacewise," Jerry observes with a deep sigh. Then he curls up tight in the fisting hammock and nods off. I can't be sure, but I think I hear a whimper. Contact. Speaking in broad gender strokes, men seek it, women withhold it. It's the essential tension that propels us biologically. And I think that's what the LPR is searching for through his extended session. In that respect, he's a lot like the client I call the Close-Getter—the guy who only wants his session in the pro dom's home, to see which brand of wheat flakes Mistress favors, what's on her bookshelf, which bills are overdue.

Maybe the marathon session, with its long hours and close confinement, is the only way for the LPR to access that greater knowledge, that intimacy and realness he so craves. In that kind of hothouse, the hair wilts and the cracks get magnified. It's like a crash course in how to be human with another person.

Like college, for example. That freshman roommate you started out hating? Meet her autistic brother, watch her try to eat pizza with the flu. You may not graduate best of friends, but guaranteed, some sort of understanding will have been reached.

6:30 a.m.: It's only a thump on a plywood door, but that *time's up* knock is like the sweet bells of heaven to my exhausted ears. Jerry rubs his eyes and comes awake, not quite believing how well he slept—"Jeez," he says, rising from the fisting hammock, "I gotta get one of these things when I move out."

Meanwhile, I'm bounding around the room like a cartoon character about to spring free of its cell. Jerry, still groggy, catches me by the arm. He just wants me to know that he had a *wonderful* time, a *truly special* experience . . . and would I like to extend the session another four hours?

QUENTIN, THE LO-FI CLIENT

In Life's Great Debate, there are certain watershed issues. You stand on one side of them or the other—no straddling allowed. Are you a Beatles person or a Stones person? Does God exist? Greater atrocity: O.J. murders or O.J. verdict?

Step into my dungeon, and here is one you'll have to answer: Does visiting a dominatrix constitute marital infidelity . . . or not?

Quentin was a longtime client of mine, a heavy bondage enthusiast who'd got his head straight about the first three of those Big Questions. Every other Thursday, we'd cue up a copy of *Sticky Fingers* and I'd tie his ass as tight as the laws of circulation permit. Then I'd stand over him, alternately taunting and teasing, as he attempted to Houdini his way free. [http://bondageu.com/campus/drbondage]

But there were a couple of months when Quentin's attendance became, well, spotty. I knew something had to be amiss. When he eventually resurfaced after an extended absence, he revealed what I'd suspected all along—an acute attack of the guilts, courtesy of Question Number Four.

So we spent the next hour, him in full rigging, trying to get to the bottom of things. Nine times out of ten, when a client does a turn-around with the speed and severity of Quentin's, there has to be a trigger. And figuring out the trigger will often lead right to the problem. In Quentin's case, it was a real no-brainer: his wife was six months pregnant with their first child, and so seeing me felt like a less-than-faithful pursuit.

At first I wasn't even going to dignify the ridiculous premise that a woman with child is somehow more "cheated on" than a woman without. Pregnancy means the demands of home and family become top priority; any decent man understands that his place is at his wife's side, ready to honor her every request—not trussed like a turkey in some dungeon across town, like a selfish, frivolous disre-specter of motherhood.

No, what gave me pause was that Quentin's moral dilemma began only when his wife started showing, and it increased right on schedule with her waistline. What that says to me is that somehow his conscience required a visual aid. Once that was revealed, I had no problem poking and prodding him until he finally confessed. The real issue here: his wife had started getting suspicious, so he'd decided to lay low with his bondage activities for the time being.

Mother's intuition or not, we had hit pay dirt. Cut-rate guilt. Not the sense of genuine regret one feels at having done someone wrong, but just the fear of being found out doing it. The dread of so-cietal disapproval; what people will think of him. What we have here is a man who's staying home not out of decent spousal loyalty but out of some piss-poor sense of obligation. An infidel, basically.

While I consider myself an old-fashioned girl, I'm no sentimen-talist. And I think that society's view of fidelity is largely informed by sentimentality. You know, that it's somehow morally superior to mate for life with one person. That sleeping around—or visiting dungeons—makes you dishonorable. To me, fidelity is about two people sticking to a contract that has been mutually agreed upon. Whatever that contract may be.

Don't get me wrong—I'm no proponent of the so-called "open relationship." I have witnessed—firsthand, regrettably—that it doesn't work. And why? Because it's a contradiction in terms, that's why. The only things it "opens" you to are bad feelings and the very worst that human nature has to offer. Disease, too. It's all way too liberated for my blood. You want to get married; *mazel tov.* You want to fuck around; stay single, stupid. So I don't think you can be a faithful mate and still play around. Conversely, however, I think it's entirely possible to be an *unfaithful* mate and never lay your hands upon another. The betraying of confidences, for instance, makes a person unfaithful, or speaking carelessly of your mate to another person. When two people become a couple, there's an implicit agreement to honorably represent each other. Bitching about your boyfriend to another guy is an insidious, passive-aggressive form of cheating. No matter what the reason, you're sending the message that the guy you're flirting with is the better man, and you wouldn't mind giving him a try.

Witness the classic mistress cliché. I don't think I need to tell you that ours is a profession that tends to attract an unusual crop of boyfriends: musicians, poets, and painters; stoners and slackers. In short, guys who can't find or keep a day job.

Now suppose you are a pro dom and you are dating one of these Romeos. Suppose you are even in love, which implies a certain contract. And because you are in love, it is downright heartbreaking to watch your fellow humping crates at Pathmark and pulling down, say, $220 for a forty-hour week. He is a brilliant, if underappreciated, electric lute player. Meanwhile, you're making that same cash in an hour or two, getting your feet rubbed and your ass kissed by some accountant who'd probably make a better mate overall. Except you shudder to think of all those free sessions you'd have to give out at bedtime.

Anyway, if Romeo is half the layabout I think he is, eventually he will lose or quit his job. And you, Mistress, will end up the patron of his art. At first it won't seem like a big deal—less pain for you to make more money, which is in keeping with the love contract.

Eventually, however, the disparity in the relationship will become ugly. Because while you will never need to worry about him sticking his dick into another—thus breaking the faithfulness clause—you will always suspect that it's only because you bought out his half of the contract. That's not fidelity, that's purchasing power. And caveat emptor: You'd have done a lot better dating that accountant—at least you'd know when your sessions begin and end. Romeo, on the other hand, has got himself a full-time submissive. You.

I don't mean to paint Quentin with the same sad brush. Fact is, he's a nice guy who seemed genuinely troubled by the notion that our biweekly bondage sessions constituted cheating on his pregnant wife. So to ease his mind a bit—I certainly wasn't going to loosen the ropes—we spent some time reexamining our definition of fidelity, culminating with this client questionnaire.

Overall, is he a good husband and provider? Does he enjoy healthy and monogamous marital relations? Is he willing to suspend our Houdini routine—gladly, without sulking—until his wife gives birth? Most of all, I'd like him to examine why he chooses to keep this side of himself away from his wife. Is there any way he can share this fantasy with *her*, not me? Fear and embarrassment do not count.

I didn't want to hear his answer. It wasn't for me to judge his fidelity. There was really only one thing I wanted to know: How in the world did his wife find out about us? After all our time together, could I have been that careless? Had I left rope burns? Lipstick stains? What?

No, he said; nothing like that. The truth was, during a week when I was away, he had seen another mistress in another dungeon. She had given him her card, this hussy, and it had fallen out of his pocket and into the sofa. His wife had found it and put it all together.

Can you imagine! Me, reverse-cuckolded by a client. That cheating slime! I couldn't wait until I saw him again. He wasn't going to wriggle out of this one so easily.

SAM I AM

In that first year of mistressing, I got to experience a pretty wide variety of clients and sessions. I'd seen everything from the garden-variety cross-dresser to the extravagant passions of the Pain-Proof Marionette Man, a guy who liked to be strung through the extremities (yes, *all* of them) with fishing wire and puppeteered from above. As with Quentin, I'd even enjoyed the occasional moral dilemma. These usually came in the form of socially unacceptable fantasies, stuff that involved race or class or inappropriate fraternizing between baby-sitters and the baby-sat.

I had a very liberal, even idealistic, attitude toward these requests. I credit my Catholic-school background for that. It seemed terribly obvious to me that what made these fantasies compelling was precisely the fact that they had been declared off-limits. That in a society so rabidly "correct," there was no way that these forbidden ideas wouldn't get linked to the sexual impulse, our greatest taboo of all. As long as the client and I understood what motivated his fantasy, and he understood its inappropriateness outside the dungeon, I saw very little reason to refuse the session.

So, in the beginning, there wasn't much that I found personally offensive. I'll admit that this was also partly due to the sheer voyeuristic thrill of hearing all these highly detailed dirty secrets. In a way, my fascination shielded me, kept me a spectator, a privileged confidante. As far as I was concerned, my actual participation was an afterthought.

But then I met up with a client, a type of client, that changed all that. In the business, this guy is known as a SAM—a Smart-Assed Masochist. This very special asshole is by far the most malignant of persons. His session, while apparently about one thing—bootlicking, caning, whatever—is really about demeaning the very mistress he professes to serve.

There are several criteria for SAMhood. They may include—but are not limited to—the following: He may be a client who purposely disobeys, to earn himself more punishment. Or maybe he asks you to change outfits three or four times, just to watch you work. He doesn't bathe or brush his teeth, just to enjoy your discomfort. He gets under your skin in the most passive-aggressive way possible, then innocently wonders what he could have done to upset you—a manipulative power-tripper of the most insidious order.

But the crowning SAM achievement is to identify your vulnerabilities, to unearth something that might really upset you—not the mistress you, but the real live person who has to live with his residue. In that respect, a SAM is truly in the eye of the beholder.

What follows are a few of their stories. Note that it was a SAM—not a pedophile, not a racist—that drove me to deploy the Angry Feminist Poetry Torture.

POETIC JUSTICE, SADIST-STYLE

We were wrestling, Irving and I, enjoying a friendly midafternoon scrap and tumble. The soothing strains of lite radio kept pulses at the low end of the FM dial. I'd been mistressing long enough to know that there was more at stake than a bruised ego or a nasty rug rash.

Perhaps we were grappling with Irving's fear of being overpowered by the fairer sex, or maybe our tussle evoked fond memories of his usual brand of foreplay. Surely these were reasons innocent enough for a forty-eight-year-old investment consultant to want to go mano a mano with the Mistress?

Distracted as he was, perhaps by a glimpse of my *Lion King* souvenir panties, I quickly gained advantage. Swinging my right leg over, I pinioned his rickety biceps beneath my six-inch stiletto heel. Careful not to pinch flesh, I raised my weight upon it; my other foot I rested lightly on his Adam's apple.

Irving's eyes darted back and forth—could it all be over this easily? I nodded gravely.

Another song came on; Nilsson's mournful warbling: "Everybody's tawkin' at me . . ."

That's when things got ugly.

Irving gurgled and gagged: the universal symbol for *time out*. But I could not let him go gracefully. He was straying from our script and, I suspected, trying to steal a peek up my skirt.

"Give me one good reason, Irv, why I should not grind you 'neath my mighty heel."

Irving gave me not one, but many. The song, you see, had brought up his suppressed memories of abuse at the hands of a girlfriend at a matinee screening of *Midnight Cowboy*. Well, not his girlfriend, actually, but a codependent woman he'd followed home from his twelve-step meeting. No, he had not been stalking her—he had only stalked the *enablers*.

Anyway, he was forced to seek validation by laying his myriad mother issues—as well as his dysfunctional fists—upon this negator. A struggle ensued, but he was not responsible for his actions. It was *she* who wanted *him*, he knew; she was just in deep denial.

"Men can be raped too," Irving gurgled tearfully. "Geraldo said so."

I increased the pressure on his throat. "Well, call an ambulance," I said, "my heart is bleeding."

What can I say? Irving forced my hand. I had no choice but to refer him to a mistress who specialized in manipulative inner-child-type scenes. Someone who could hog-tie him with his own line of shit so expertly that he'd spend his session listening to her detail her own agonizing memories. And if I knew this mistress, later, he'd wind up apologizing for making her dredge them up in the first place.

So I gave Irving the number of this dominatrix I know—I'll call her Patsy—who was the self-proclaimed Victim of Everything. It seems that at the precise moment of her birth, God, that chauvinist, realigned the planets directly against her, leaving her a hapless pawn in the mind fucks perpetrated by society in general, the evil penis wielders in particular.

In Patsy's universe—of which she was the paranoid center—all sex was rape, either at the moment or, usually, in retrospect, because patriarchal brainwashing had rendered her incapable of asserting herself horizontally.

In a similar way, all employment was gender-based exploitation. If you ever thought that having to work was just a generally lousy fact of life, to Patsy it was a blatant corporate plot to keep her down. Imagine a man paying a measly eight dollars an hour for her hunt-and-peck skills and then oppressing her by asking that she leave her go-go boots at home and refrain from using the office equipment for her personal work.

"I bet Mr. ——— wouldn't look at me like that if I were a man!" was an oft-repeated exclamation of Patsy's. Yes, Patsy, but I bet that if you were a man you wouldn't have left twenty-seven copies of your latest writings, *My Cunt Runneth Over,* in the Xerox machine.

I met Patsy at the dawn of the nineties, when her suppressed childhood memories began to rise from their rotting cribs. Coincidentally, these demons surfaced just in time to compete with the demands of early adulthood: get a job, find an apartment, purchase your own toilet paper.

Not so coincidentally, her inability to find a workplace that welcomed sequined cleavage (she had the clothes long before her tenure as a dominatrix) left her with plenty of free afternoons to enjoy the Golden Age of Self-Disclosure TV. So on my sofa she sat, chain-smoking and throwing her tarot cards, nursing these mewling childhood kittens on the tit of Oprah and Sally Jesse and Geraldo.

Every day she grew stronger in her belief that the abuse she had suffered in childhood—real or imagined, and imagine the atrocities she was suppressing!—had encoded her forever as a victim. It was therefore her destiny to walk through life—just as she had walked through several past lives—seeking abusers; it was the only way she knew. Long-distance phone calls to her psychic—a forty-one-year-old alcoholic recluse—corroborated this theory.

So how was poor Patsy to navigate the cold, murky waters of adulthood? By attaching herself like a barnacle to someone else's ship, that's how. Someone who would understand that the world had so betrayed her that she, as Patsy's friend, would never take advantage of her vulnerable state by causing her any more grief. Things that might cause Patsy grief were:

1. Request that she get her dead ass off the sofa and find a job. No, that might remind Patsy too much of her mother, who was both smothering and demanding and had once forced her to baby-sit before she was ready to handle it.
2. Suggest, in a nonjudgmental fashion, that she might people her poetry with things other than eyes and mirrors, souls and smiles that sighed and cried and died and ate apple pie. Are you trying to stifle her creativity?! The precise reason she left home in the first place, and if you were half a friend you'd know that.
3. Intimate that perhaps it was just a tad, ahem, unhealthy that the two of you spend so much time together, and wouldn't she like to cultivate some other friends? Well, I think you know enough about Patsy to guess that this is when the waterworks begin. And *then* what do you do?

I'll tell you what I did—I fell all over myself apologizing to this freeloader when I should have been evicting her, and running around town trying to find a take-out entrée that didn't remind her of all those gut-wrenching dysfunctional family dinners and resenting every minute of it. Meanwhile, she was back at my house, talking long-distance to her psychic, who had just gotten the vibe that I was once Patsy's executioner during the Spanish Inquisition.

Okay, so you don't need to be Nostradamus to see that this friendship was going to end badly. The day I presented Patsy with the Final Notice phone bill was the day I joined her pantheon of abusers. I may have lost access to a swell pair of go-go boots, but I sure regained ownership of my apartment pretty quickly. Patsy, equipped with more self-preservation skills than an Outward Bound alumnus, soon found herself another meal ticket, and I hear their phone has been shut off permanently.

And then, Patsy got angry. Angry for all the past evils that life had dealt her, and even a few that life hadn't. I received volumes of anonymous poetry in the mail, informing me that my eyes were mere mirrors of betrayal, my smile a lie full of razors that slashed at her soul, which had heretofore been open wide as a flying vagina. Or something like that.

They weren't bad poems, really, except that their ballistic intent was undermined by the fact that she couldn't seem to locate the caps key on her typewriter. I could only assume that the style was either an indication of her "lowercase" feelings toward me, or that I was getting hate mail from e. e. cummings.

And as Patsy's anger grew, so did her body hair. Crotch hair, leg hair, armpit hair, all grew to lengths certain to inform society that patriarchal standards of beauty meant nothing to her. She began to embrace—no, tackle—a brand of feminism that has always baffled me, and I've let a few razors rust in my day, I assure you.

You know what I'm talking about: that man-bad/woman-good manifesto. I am a strong woman, you are a weak man. I want no part of you. Except for my boyfriend, whom I will ridicule and dissect, as I wait patiently by the phone for his call.

I own my body and no one can tell me what to do with it. This gives me license to tell other women—such as strippers, center-folds, and entertainers—exactly what they should do with theirs, because they can't possibly know what they want.

I am a woman on my own terms. That is why I will modify my appearance to directly oppose the male aesthetic. If they like high heels, I will wear Birkenstocks. If it's flowing tresses that they favor, I will shave my head. See? No man is going to tell me what to do!

Above all, I will have no sense of humor whatsoever. That would imply that I endorse the absurdities and complexities of life. Worse, it might cause me to accidentally entertain a viewpoint less rigid than my own. [http://no-men-allowed.com/directory/grrl-web/Girly]

Believe me, I've devoted many hours trying to make sense of Patsy's version of feminism. The only thing I can conclude is that it was invented by a man who truly despises women, and would like us to live lives of misery and ugly footwear.

But Patsy does have one special mistressing skill, a punishment more brutal than anything I could have devised for Irving. I personally have seen it render grown men prostrate with anguish, begging for the sweet release that only death can bring. Due to its extreme savagery, I was bound by conscience to save it as an absolute last resort. But here it is, that most grueling of ordeals, the Angry Feminist Poetry Torture.

Irving is hustled into a darkened room. Immediately, a pitcher of lukewarm espresso is forced down his throat by a mistress who deftly picks his pocket—espressos don't come cheap, you know. Then he is strapped to an undersized, wobbly metal stool by another mistress, who proceeds to elbow him and step all over his feet. A few minutes elapse during which the two attending mistresses refuse to speak to him no matter what he says. Rather, they communicate their feelings for him with glares and exaggerated tongue clucking. His very existence is an emblem of their oppression!

Soon enough, all that caffeine begins galloping through his system like the Four Horsemen of the Apocalypse. His colonic discomfort is multiplied as one mistress shoves a fist-sized butt plug up his ass. To muffle his cries, a handful of superabsorbent tampons are stuffed into his mouth.

The mistresses nestle close on either side of Irving, but if one of his knees should come in contact with one of theirs—watch out! Irving gets a swift kick in the scrotum. Then, as the mistresses blow clove-cigarette smoke into Irving's nostrils, the lights come up, and that's when the fun really begins.

Into the dungeon stomps Mistress Patsy, in combat boots, cutoff shorts, and a plaid flannel shirt tied at the tits to artfully reveal her oppressed navel. Wielding a five-pound notebook, unlined yet teeming with angry, sophomoric testaments to her fury, she crouches so close that Irving is nearly sucked into the two-car garage of Patsy's flaring nostrils.

Patsy is gender privileged to shove her bosom right under his nose, as if to taunt his inner rapist. As the tampon strings in his mouth tickle her cleavage, the other two mistresses strike up the chorus: *What are you looking at?! What are you looking at?!* But this is a trick, Irving, so be warned! If he should dare to eye the wall of flesh looming before him, he is instantly and brutally clobbered with the five-pound notebook. Hard enough to stun, but not enough to slip him into merciful unconsciousness as she farts out her diatribe at point-blank range: *MY VICTIMIZED VAGINA CRIES THE EYES AND LIES OF YOUR PATRIARCHAL SOCI-ETY. . . .*

And so on, for as long as it takes for Irving to admit that his penis is indeed the root of all evil. And if she should run out of poems first, there's always that guitar. Cruel and inhuman punishment? You be the judge. Me, I prefer to think of it as poetic justice, sadist-style.

CUCKOLDING THE LILLIPUD

Madame Defarge was Lady Leona's godmother; she had managed to survive New York City for the last twenty years with command of a single English phrase: "Black bangs bring out the eyes," which she used often, to ominous effect. Moled and mustached, she looked like a real pro at the maiden-aunty arts: poultice making, tick removing, the vanquishing of unclean spirits—that sort of thing. During the day, she worked the wig counter at Bloomies; nights, she baby-sat the dominatrices of Lady Leona's Reformatory. In both places, her pet phrase served her equally well.

We called her Madame Defarge because the kindly old bat was constantly, nervously, knitting something—the names of her enemies, our names—we presumed. And, like the Dickens character, her pastime was nothing more than a cover for her true mission: making sure we didn't rob Leona blind when Leona was out schmucking certain other "specialty clients" blind.

But something must've gotten lost in the translation when Leona outlined her job duties to Madame Defarge. Rather than policing us,

Defarge seemed to actually aid and abet our cause. She remained blissfully ignorant, installed (actually, *locked*) in Leona's office as we snuck client after client past her, keeping the entire take—Leona's half plus ours. I remember one late night in particular, right around Labor Day, when the scamming was beginning to reach critical mass. I'd arrived late for work—punctuality was no longer an issue, under the Defarge regime—and walked straight into some major dungeon intrigue.

The stink of money hung in the air, mingled with the scent of disinfectant and Shalimar, Defarge's signature aroma. And one man's aftershave, pungent and keening, the kind you might associate with foreign discotheques and gold-tone chest medallions.

They had the guy in lockup in Dungeon #3 for a full two hours before I got a crack at him. Whatever they were doing in there, it was exhausting the girls at a rate of two per hour. They came spiraling out of the room, one by one, tight of jaw, chain-smoking Kools, and spluttering incoherently. And dropping rolled-up, powdered fifties as they walked.

Okay, so you didn't need a masters in pharmacology to figure that the guy was blowing his brains out—but that was nothing new to us. There had to be a catch, and I needed to know what it was. "He's into the rude," muttered one of the girls. Then she scurried into the lounge, where the doms were wearily passing around a bottle of warm Champale, too spent to count their money.

I steeled myself and entered Dungeon #3. The room was like an inexpertly mirrored sauna, thick with mentholated steam. Through all the smoke and stink I saw a huge pile of white powder laid out atop the punishment horse. I scooped up a fingernail and touched it to my tongue. Clorox.

This was a valuable piece of information. A rich guy with large quantities of shitty drugs has got to be a sucker. He'd obviously been taken before; now it was my turn.

I squinted through the smog and eyed my prey. A thick-bodied Arab guy, roasted brown as a chestnut, lay supine on the bondage table. Not unattractive; even his less than model-perfect features—hawk nose, tar-black pelt of chest hair—seemed to smack of wealth, insouciance, and excessive appetites. From where I stood, it was hard to imagine what his problem might be.

Slowly, lazily, he helped himself to a hefty line with an extralong pinkie nail. "So tell me . . ." he said finally, "what do you think of my penis?" I thought about it, long and hard. If you know anything about the effects of cocaine upon male prowess, you understand that there is no pun intended.

Fact is, penis questions are generally trick questions; the astute mistress knows that there is a right answer and a wrong one and is loath to tip her hand until she's sure which is which. "Don't waste my time," I replied, taking a seat between him and his stash.

He lit a menthol cigarette. "It is small, don't you think?"

"It is the most minuscule thing," I said with great conviction, "that I have ever seen."

He nodded evenly and handed me a rolled-up fifty. I wasn't sure if this meant I was being offered the money or the drugs, but I'll be damned if some slave's gonna order me to get high. So I pocketed the bill and went into my standard mistress dick-dissing spiel: *You've got some nerve bringing that miserable stack o' dimes in here, Lilliput Boy—what, do you jerk off with tweezers?!* Et cetera.

I ran with that for a while as he listened attentively, snorkeling lines, carefully considering each insult. When I had used up all known synonyms for "pencil dick," I took one of his menthols and lit it.

"This cigarette is like Long Dong Silver compared to you," I said. (What can I tell you? Sometimes you've got to use whatever's handy.)

"That is why you fucked my friend, no?"

A-hah! I thought—*now we're getting somewhere.* "That is why I fucked your friend, and some you never even knew about," I said.

"But mostly it was my friends, no?"

"Almost without exception, yes."

"Why don't you tell me all about it," he asked. "I want you should say the details I not already know."

And so it began, the session that had taken me a full half-hour to figure out. He lay there, snorting coke and serenely masturbating as I regaled him with myriad tales of his cuckolding: a steamy encounter with his best man, Emir, in the bathroom, a quickie with Rasul—his business partner—on the office Xerox machine.

Mostly, my dear Arab friend seemed to enjoy the pleasures I'd stolen when he was nearby, such as the time I'd bedded Omar and Ahmed—his soccer pals—while he was eating couscous on the patio.

But don't expect me to supply *you* with the sordid specifics—this unrepentant tart tends to blank out such details—and besides, I doubt you're prepared to bless me with as many fifties as Cheat Boy did. Plus, once we got rolling, he was a great help, asking questions that would heighten the seediness and scandal: "And what was I doing when you were with Emir? And did you crawl into my bed right after? And how many times did such-and-such happen? And how did that make you feel?"

I'll tell you how it made me feel—not like a dominatrix at all. It reminded me of this guy I used to go out with—we had what they call an "open" relationship—who used to love to hear tell of my extracurricular activities. No, I mean he really, really loved to hear about such things—the stories became our sex life.

Soon enough, I began to realize that it wasn't his way of celebrating my sexual independence, but rather his way of saying he didn't really care about me or anything that I did.

When I applied this reasoning to my client, what I came up with was a guy who needed to keep his woman in a place where he didn't have to care about her. His buddies were his people and women were the evil outsiders best passed around like a warm bottle of Champale.

Typical macho-dick posturing; I'm aware that it exists, no big deal. The trouble is that this guy needed *me* to underscore this point, and it left me feeling like some squinty-eyed pervert had just rubbed

up against me in a crowded subway car. Worse, he'd managed to res-
urrect a couple of my own unpleasant memories in the process.
I can't speak for my coworkers, but for me, that's what was so exhausting about the encounter. When our time was up, I had no problem tapping him for a nice fat tip. "Gimme two hundred bucks," I
said. "I need to buy a really fancy, slutty dress."

"Is that the dress that Adnan is going to hoist up around your
shoulders when he takes you in the hold of my motorboat?"

"No, it's the dress *you're* going to wear when all of my girlfriends come in here and stick a really large bat up your ass," I
replied sweetly.

Loverboy left soon after that. And I was left with a sad, sinister
feeling about everything. I even felt bad about what we'd been
doing to Defarge, hustling behind her back. It seemed like the whole
world came down to people taking things from one another—drugs,
money, dignity, goodwill.

I retreated to the office to check on the old lady. I expected to find
her nodded off, like she usually was at this hour. But she was wide
awake, and deep into her knitting. We sat in utter silence; I held her
yarn as she stitched the collar onto a teal blue merino wool sweater.
"What a scumbag, that guy," she said, in perfect, unaccented English. "How do you like my sweater?"

FRANKLIN THE MILLIONAIRE

MONEYTRIPPER

So we're sitting around the dungeon one Rosh Hashanah like a bunch of spinster sadists, broke and dejected. Business was so dead it was as if the hand of God Himself had reached down from the heavens and snipped the phone lines. Giddy from hunger, I splurged and bought a ninety-nine-cent three-pack of those Korean-deli fig Newtons, the kind with the seeds that get stuck in the dental work for weeks. If I was lucky, I thought, a few might dislodge and provide welcome sustenance in the lean High Holy Days to come.

"Wouldn't it be nice," said Mistress J., "if some guy just walked in here, I mean, just walked *right through that door*, gave us money, and split?" J. is a bit of a simpleton and poorer than all of us combined, so we indulged her, murmuring polite agreement, turning away with our scowls. Then, like an audiovisual aid, Franklin appeared at the door.

A dungeon legend, Franklin had a money fetish. Simply put, he was a filthy-wealthy speed freak who got off on the exchanging of the green. I personally had never seen him, but I'd heard the rumors: he only wore Armani suits, and only once, discarding them like Kleenex after each use. His session consisted of inventing a series of odd tasks for his mistress for which he would tip the big bucks. "Spit in my face for fifty dollars. . . . Kick me in the ass for the contents of my back pocket. . . . Pin me down for two minutes, this C-note is yours. . . ." And so on. In short, he ran mistresses ragged but richer.

Then there was his grand finale, where he would stuff a $30 dress sock with money and stick it up his ass. This sock might contain any amount from $20 to $1,000; it was yours for the taking. And you were expected to extract it by any means necessary.

This was nothing more than dungeon hearsay until I was face-to-face with him in Dungeon #2. Ferret-faced and tweaking, he stood stripped down to a pair of silk boxers which, I noted, probably cost more than I had earned in the last three weeks. A leather purse, stuffed with crisp, unused hundreds—the new counterfeit-proof kind—rested atop the punishment horse.

What a despicable weasel, I thought to myself. He stroked the leather purse like a well-fed pet. "It's so nice to finally make your acquaintance," I said.

And then it began, a flurry of deeds and reckonings, fifties and twenties, credits and debits. "I'll give you a hundred dollars," he said, "if you can punch me so hard that I see stars."

I picked up a crumpled twenty that had fallen out of my bra. "But how will I know if you see stars?"

"You'll just have to trust me."

So I hauled off and punched him square in the jaw—more tentatively than I was feeling, but I wasn't sure it would be fiscally prudent to bloody my new meal ticket. "Well . . . ?" I said as he rubbed his stubbly chin.

"I can't rightly say as I saw stars," he countered. "More like an asteroid, maybe—and that's only worth twenty."

Now I was pissed. "Oh yeah? What's the Milky Way going for these days?" And before I could even think I clocked him, hard—I mean, really hard—in the groin with the tip of my shoe. What can I say? It was reflex.

He doubled over and did an entire little pain jig while I stood there thinking, *Oh Mary Help of Christians, shit, shit, shit, don't make me call an ambulance, Amen.*

But Franklin recovered. In fact, he looked up at me with an expression of utter and superior contentment. "I think I'm in love," he said.

I sighed with relief.

"And when I am in love I'll spend so much money on my mistress, you won't even believe it. Why, just last week I gave Mistress Sondra sixteen hundred just to walk across my back. Is that crazy or what? Am I not one fucked-up crazy person?"

I shrugged and held out my hand. "Can we safely assume that stars were seen? Huh?"

"Mmmm. Big stars. Constellations."

"Well, then ante the hell up."

"Can I get you later? Don't you trust me?"

"I trust you just fine. Now pay me."

"Oh, I see . . ." he said. "This is all about the money to you, right? That's all you're in this for." He eyed me speculatively, like he knew what I looked like naked and tied up.

"Shove your money up your ass," I said. Given the nature of all that I'd heard about him, it seemed like a good middle-of-the-road retort.

The session deteriorated rapidly from there. And I'd say this downward spiral had nothing to do with the fact that I'd so savagely knocked him in the nuts, but because he had pinpointed the moment that the greed frenzy transported me. Now he had me, and he was done just as sure as if he had jizzed all over me. When it was over, I felt dirty and cheap—and not in a good way, either. Also $240 richer.

But what's the starting salary for pride swallowing? Dignity abandonment?

What bothered me about Franklin's session is what bothers me about all moneytrippers and their sessions. It's just an uglier form of what we call "topping from the bottom," where the slave is really calling all the shots. Guys like Franklin pimp our poverty. They get hard-ons watching the hungry cash register in a mistress's eyes. They come in when business is slow and exploit the buyer's market—which is probably not dissimilar to the way they made their fortunes in the first place. It's not that I'm a tree-hugging anticapitalist. You made your money fair and square—or maybe not—you wanna enjoy it, more power to you. The problem is that the way these guys enjoy their money is by rubbing your face in it—*don't you wish you were rich like me?*—because none of their money has ever bought them anything of value.

And that's why Franklin's session left me in such a snit. Because even with my $240, I felt cheated; during the course of our frenzied encounter he had actually run a tab of over $1,700.

Yes, I'd been mistressing long enough to realize it was not necessarily a real figure. It was part of his fantasy. But I also knew what kind of improvements that $1,700 could have made in my life at that time—and it was a damned sight more than a new set of silk boxer shorts, I assure you.

Franklin knew that too, and he wanted to see what he could get for it. Not that he expected any kind of sexual favors—these guys are often asexual anyway, being so hopped up on greed (and speed). No, his satisfaction came from mocking my aspirations and slapping me with a sense of futility.

Once Franklin had put a price on my head, I knew he would someday return. And I knew he would try the sock-up-his-ass trick. In a perfect world, I'd just tell him to keep his shitty money. Except that he'd probably make sure to time his visit for the Chanukah/Christmas lull. That way, I'd be broke again, and I'd really have to think about it.

PART II

THE LIFESTYLE

THE MATRICULATED MISTRESS

How do you know when mistressing is no longer a lark, but a career? Take this simple quiz:

- Has Windex, Armor All, or saddle soap replaced Cheer as your primary detergent?
- Does "eyebrow maintenance" mean drawing them on, rather than tweezing?
- If yes, can you sketch in your brows with precision, without being mistaken for a Picasso?
- Do you expect men to address you as "Ma'am," or "Goddess"? If they don't, are there consequences?
- Can you untangle twenty-five feet of rope from a public washing machine with ease and dignity, even in front of six curious neighbors?
- Do you presume that most businessmen wear women's panties beneath their trousers? How about stockings? A butt plug?
- Have you ever accidentally given your mistress name when it

just wasn't appropriate? "Hi, I'm Chaotica. You must be Bobby's parents!"

If you answered "yes" to two or more of the above, it's time to face facts. You are no longer taking a little walk on the wild side; you have officially set up shop there.

I'd been mistressing for almost a year when I realized that it had been ages since I'd dusted off my résumé, much less dragged my ass to a job interview. At first, I was a little scandalized—was I blowing years of education, of promise, on diapering grown men? Shouldn't I be in an office, making them coffee, rather than in Dungeon #1, making them lick my shoes?

This delusion fizzled out pretty quickly. The truth was, even if I weren't working at Leona's, there was little chance I'd be in any kind of résumé situation. Instead, I'd be writing, like I already was, and trying to land some kind of regular column in a magazine or newspaper—like I already had. The only difference was that without my dungeon income, freelancing would be lo-fi and painfully shabby. No cool clothes, no foot rubs, just the soul-crushing demoralization of ramen noodles and bargain-basement shopping. It was just not my style.

And I had one more compelling incentive. Working in the dungeon forced me to focus on writing in a way that no "respectable" job ever could. I knew in my heart that a straight nine-to-fiver would only make me lazy, complacent—just collecting a paycheck would make it easy to pretend that I had something to show for myself. Throw in a 401(k) and a dental plan, and I'd feel like a goddamned prodigy.

Being a dominatrix, however, meant that I had absolutely *nothing* to show for myself! This I found liberating, even inspirational. Pitted against the seediness, the stigma, the sheer aimlessness of the underworld, the good Catholic girl in me finally had a reason to prove herself. If I wasn't writing about it, how else could I justify nosing around the inferno?

Still, I promised myself that there was no way I'd go another year—nay, another minute—in the dungeon unless I was absolutely cool with it, as a mistress and as a chronicler of mistressing. So I stayed at the dungeon, but it was different. After a year, I'd seen all I was going to see. If I wanted any new S&M experiences, I'd have to move on to another level, visit the hardcore clubs or seek out the serious pain mavens, the lifestylers. Or I could specialize in something, like cross-dressing or wrestling, or Japanese bondage—the S&M equivalent of declaring a major.

But none of this appealed to me at all. The truth was that while I wasn't learning anything new about S&M—nor did I care to expand my repertoire—I was becoming really good at just *being* a mistress.

And so the *lifestyle* of mistressing, the arcana of the job, became my field of study. I wanted to document this rarefied slice of twentieth-century living, how the everyday played out in our dungeon biosphere, and why the rules and the etiquette were only amplified versions of the more traditional workplace. That it required a dual identity, and that sometimes these worlds collided—this only sweetened the research.

RUBY, PHONE HOMO

There I was, chatting on the Lesbo Line in the middle of a Tuesday afternoon. Even though I was new to phone sex, I think you'll agree that I was getting the hang of it pretty quickly.

"So, like, uh . . . what are you wearing?" I murmur into Lady Leona's pink princess phone.

"A . . . very . . . sexy . . . outfit."

"Is it really sexy?" I ask. "Can you tell me what it looks like, exactly?"

"It . . . makes . . . me . . . soooo . . . hot," she replies. She's a wet-and-ready college coed; she majors in hot.

"Can I ask you something, Misty Bleu?"

"Ask . . . me . . . anything."

"Ask her to take off all her clothes!" hisses Chester the Molester, jacking off furiously into one of my old school socks.

"Is Misty your actual name, or is it something more regular, like Mary? Did your parents—the Bleus?—worry that you were gonna grow up to be a phone-sex operator if they named you Misty?"

Misty giggles and lets a long silence pass. She's burning up the minutes for both of us, and God love her for it. Together we're giving a whole new meaning to the term "friend-on-the-other-end."

"Why . . . don't . . . you . . . tell . . . me . . . what . . . *you're* . . . wearing?" Misty says finally. "And please—don't . . . leave . . . *anything* . . . out."

I'm sitting on Lady Leona's sectional sofa in pigtails and my old plaid school uniform, pretending to be something other than my jaded, world-weary self. Meanwhile, Chester the Molester, my very own Humbert Humbert, lustily spurs me to new depths of depravity.

Chester, you'll recall, is the guy who likes to corrupt the *Barely Legal* set via bad porn and today's specialty, 900 numbers. And before you pass judgment on the statutory implications of this scene, remember that at twenty-five, I'm Barely Believable.

Chester snatches the phone from me and cups the mouthpiece with his non-jack-off hand. "Twenty minutes have passed," he complains, "and we haven't even seen her tits yet!"

I nod compassionately. This Misty chick is good. And slow. At $3.95 a minute, she makes Forrest Gump on a handful of roofies sound glib as a carnival barker.

"So . . ." I begin slowly, "why . . . don't . . . you . . . take . . . off . . . your . . . clothes . . . for . . . me?"

This had all started about a week before, right after my last visit with Chester. As he was dropping me back at the dungeon, he inquired as to the status of my cherry. I figured, what the hell, he already believes I'm eighteen, may as well go for it. Fully in character, I managed to blush prettily and confide that, as a matter of fact, no, I had never known the pleasures of carnal love with a man.

"I thought that might be the case," Chester leered, stroking his erection through a spent pair of fishnet stockings, the ones he wore only in the car.

Blame it on hubris, but I just couldn't leave well enough alone. No, I had to go and mention that although I had never actually done it with a guy, there was this girl back in high school, and we had, you know, tried stuff together. "It's like, with a girl, I feel a lot safer."

"And, probably, a lot hotter," Chester noted. "How about we get together next Tuesday, and I'll have a big surprise for you."

The surprise turned out to be a stack of girl-on-girl porn. Girls with strap-ons, girls without. Girls who peed on other girls and girls who drank the pee; shy girls and anal girls and leather girls; girls gang-banging girls. All of this was just a warm-up for the main event, my pricey little phone date with Misty Bleu. As far as I could tell, Chester's goal was to get me so frenzied with cunt lust that I would pleasure myself right then and there, never minding that he was looking on. He would then offer to lend a hand—or two—and we would segue into other pursuits.

Now, I think we all know that the chances of me spontaneously masturbating in front of Chester were roughly the same as the chances of me spontaneously combusting. My goal was to get through this encounter without giving anything up, but still keeping Chester interested enough to see me again. Misty Bleu's goal, meanwhile, was pretty much the same. And so there existed between us an unspoken agreement that we would help each other tough it out, two sisters-in-arms, so that we could both go the hell home and live to work another day.

So I sit there fiddling with some stray elastic threads from my waistband and let Misty grind out her stock Lesbian First Encounter story. Just last summer, Misty and her friend Tammi did one of those Hedonism II tour packages in order to party and, you know, meet some guys. When they got to their room, they discovered that they were stuck with one king-size bed.

You know those Hedonism places, they ply you with tropical drinks of every frozen hue, and it wasn't long before Tammi got drunk and brought her paragliding instructor, Dirk, back to their room. But Misty had retired early. Dirk touched Tammi; Tammi touched Dirk. Tammi touched Misty, accidentally, of course, waking her up partly. Misty, confused by sleep, touched back. And then, though they pretended it was an accident, things took a more purposeful turn . . .

"Ask her if she's touching herself yet!" Chester butts in. I press the receiver to my chest and throw him a look of weary disdain. I've done my best to relay all the juicy parts as Misty recites them; still he insists on being this backseat masturbator. And, anyway, I've got my own questions I'd like Misty Bleu to answer.

I'd like to know how old she really is, and how she got into doing the phone-sex thing. Is she reclining comfortably on a couch, or must she sit upright in a rolling metal chair in some six-by-six cubby, tethered to her post by a headset? Is she allowed to leave the place for lunch, or must she order in? How much of that $3.95 per minute is hers to take home? How many Chesters must she verbally jerk off before she can pay her own phone bill?

Mostly, I'd like her to tell me how she manages to keep that healthy, sanity-saving separation between the fantasy aspect of her job and the reality of her own sex life. Does she even have a sex life? And, if she does, what happens when her partner asks her to talk dirty to him/her? Does it make her feel like she's at work?

Has a client ever said anything to her that made her feel filthy and cheap and less than human? Conversely, has anyone ever said something that got her really aroused? Aroused enough to actually touch herself like she tells me she's doing?

Hah! you say—now I'm thinking like twisted old Chester. Not true. I'm thinking like any normal human being with my experience might, given the circumstances. It's Chester's influence, his need to turn every sexual impulse into an opportunity for exploitation, that's making it seem dirty.

So I place the phone down on Lady Leona's beveled glass coffee table. But I don't hang up, out of consideration for Misty—I'm sure she has bills to pay. I tell Chester that this phone business simply isn't my bag—if I'm going to explore my latent bisexuality, I'm going to have to do it with a real person, face-to-face. "Perhaps that can be arranged," Chester purrs. "Perhaps there's a special friend you'd like to play with us?"

With Misty listening in, I tell Chester that yes, I do have a girl-friend for whom I have certain . . . feelings. And I've always thought that she might be receptive, if only she were given the proper incentive.

Chester's all over that like a sauce. "Well, maybe she can come up here next time and play with us," he begins. "And I can do my crazy thing"—he waves his hand to indicate his girlie movies, his kneesock-encased erection, and me—"and then afterward, when I'm gone, you can take her aside and say, 'Gee, wasn't that disgusting? Aren't you glad we're both girls together, not gross like him?'" Chester begins to lose himself in the reverie. "And then from there," he gasps, "you can get right into her tight little snatch!"

Sometimes I think the funniest things are also the saddest and most true. Misty Bleu must be having a similar thought. From the receiver, I hear a genuine laugh. No girlie giggle, but a woman's earthy cackle, the laugh of a fellow sex soldier. And this time, nobody's faking nothing.

MISTRESS, MAY I?

An old client of mine, Manny, resurfaced after a six-month dis-appearance. This caused me some concern because I used to see him two, three times a month. I missed our sessions: me blowing noxious plumes of smoke into his face at point-blank range, bitch-ing him out, stream-of-consciousness style, and grinding a very sharp, long stiletto heel into his crotch as if snuffing out a cigarette. Ah, but we had ourselves a merry old time.

When we were done, I asked him where he'd been for the last half year. He is a sweet little submissive and he didn't want to offend me, so I really had to crowbar it out of him. Finally, he confessed that he had come in for a session one day when I was unavailable, and was informed he would have to have his session with a certain Mistress X, as conniving and humorless a harridan as I have ever met. Apparently, she'd railroaded him into his least-favorite room and force-fed him someone else's session, which had absolutely nothing to do with why he was there.

But Manny endured—what choice did he have? She had him scared shitless. And Mistress X went on to forbid him to see anyone else at Lady Leona's except for her, warning him that she would find out if he even attempted it.

Needless to say, I was appalled. I asked him why he, a successful and intelligent gentleman, would put up with this type of fascism. Didn't he realize that it was his dime, his session, and ultimately his ass that he was handing over to this evil beast?

"Well," he replied simply, "this isn't my game, and I don't know the rules." And Manny waved his arms about as if to indicate Dungeon #3, Lady Leona's establishment, even the entire commercial S&M scene in New York City.

So this one's for all you submissive men who'd like to try a session with a professional mistress but are either scared or baffled as to how to behave and what to expect.

I'm going to skip right over the part about you showing up for your session on time, with sincere intent, and clean. That is, if you're just in it to gawk and walk, please don't waste our time; if you want to see what the interior of a bondage parlor looks like, try Hellfire or the Vault, two popular clubs. Some dungeons charge a small "consultation fee" just to walk in the door.

And did I say I wasn't going to talk hygiene? Well, I lied. It's of paramount importance that your body is fresh and clean. You wouldn't want to waste valuable session time trotting off to the rest room with a bar of soap in your mouth—or in any other orifice deemed hygienically deficient—would you? By the same token, this being the age of AIDS, hepatitis, and cooties, you have every right to inquire about the health measures employed by the dungeon you visit. Any place that won't tell you how and how often they sterilize the implements, won't provide condoms for covering gags and other tools of destruction, as well as latex gloves for handling whatever and underpads to come between you and other surfaces, is a place you should exit immediately.

Fortunately, most dungeons recognize high health standards as a modern-day selling point, and are often more conscientious than you yourself might be. Oh, and feel free to request double-bagging—that is, doubling up on whatever safety shield you might be using. Latex gloves are pennies apiece.

Let's talk about meeting the dom of your dreams. You have the right to meet all the mistresses who are available for sessions when you arrive. They'll most likely sit you down in a room and come in to meet you, one by one. If you really want to get things off on the wrong foot, be sure to be bare-assed naked when they enter the room, setting your hairy fruit bowl down somewhere you weren't invited. We absolutely bristle at such presumption. So let's agree not to do that, okay?

Here come the dominas, and aren't they exquisite? But please don't fawn or gawk—save that for the actual session. A respectful meeting of the gaze is appreciated; a firm, dry handshake. Inform each domina of the alias you'll be using—John, Mark, Steve, or David seem to be the most popular—and listen closely when the mistress introduces herself. Repeat the name for better retention; file away a connecting image so you won't forget. If she says, "Hello, I am Svetlana," you think *Svetlana, Ice Hellion of the Forbidden Baltic.* Works like a charm. While you're at it, do your best to remember the phony name you gave yourself.

Ask each mistress what her area of expertise is. This part is best kept brief. Understand that you have the power to trigger a thermonuclear war in the mistress lounge should one girl accuse another of lingering too long and trying to "steal" the session. Do not abuse this power.

Once you've decided whom you'd like to see, you'll get a more in-depth consultation. You will also get to see all the available rooms and decide which one is best equipped for your particular passion.

And speaking of passions: you know what you like, so be as specific as possible. You're not doing us any favors by making us read your mind or ungag you midstream so that you can confide that, well, you have a deep and abiding fear of being gagged.

You have the right to ask the mistress to don the fetish gear most fitting to your interests, as well as a costume, if the mistress has it, for certain types of role playing. But mind your p's and q's, *por favor.* You're not ordering a Chinese combo meal; this is a human being you're conversing with. Piss us off in the beginning and things have a way of . . . evening out.

Which brings me to a very important point. Up to this juncture, you can expect your mistress to be polite, businesslike, and thorough. Arch, maybe, and with a hint of the attitude to come, sure, but know this: abuse begins and ends in the session. It shouldn't have started yet—if it has, you may be dealing with a rank amateur or an asshole, a dom who doesn't know when to turn it on, off, or up. And her understanding of what's acceptable will loom much larger when you're at her complete mercy, take my word for it. This is your chance to turn back or ask to see another.

Also, this is the time to discuss clearly how much pain you can take, and whether or not we can leave marks. Trust me, we don't want your wife to find grill bars branded on your ass either. We like your business, and we want you to come back.

Then there's Verbal: how you'd like to be spoken to—how severely, how specifically. Would you like her to humiliate you for what you're doing, or for who you are—your genuine human idiosyncrasies? Remember also that there needn't be any patter at all. You two can simply hang around and chat like two pals, one flogging the flying shit out of the other.

Finally, let's talk some very basic money matters. The cash you fork over is never referred to as a "fee" or "payment." Polite people call it a "tribute" or "gift," as if to make it sound voluntary. Some people seem to think that this semantic sleight of hand will somehow keep us out of trouble with the IRS and local authorities. I have yet to understand why. But you know the burnout folklore that says if you ask an undercover cop if he's a cop, he has to say yes? Well, this is the same kind of delusion.

In any case, the tribute for an S&M session is intended to cover the time spent, not the activity enjoyed. So don't let some enterprising young hussy con you into believing that there's some kind of "lipstick fee" involved in a cross-dressing session, or an "extra rope" tariff for big-and-tall bondage lovers. If you've managed to come up with some fantasy so extravagant and over the top that it justifies a surcharge, expect to hear about it up front, when you have the right to decide how you'd like to proceed.

Some places, if you ask nicely, will sometimes allow you to have another mistress make a ten-to-twenty-minute cameo appearance during your session. We have every confidence that you will present her with some kind of lovely incentive to make it worth her while. You can look to your main mistress for guidance here.

Also, as long as you don't actually utter that little word that rhymes with *whips*—you know, To Insure Prompt Suffering—the conventional wisdom is yes, absolutely. It's not mandatory, it's not always even expected, and you won't get hurt if you don't ante up. Being a cheap dickhead is really your own cross to bear. But I've never seen anyone turn one down.

As for gifts—an item of some sort, like some kind of S&M doohickey, flowers, or caviar—that's really not something that will help put your mistress through grad school. Presents are nice, but woe, woe to the submissive who presents me with a piece of lingerie or a sex toy. You keep a respectful distance, pal. Do I want you thinking of me in some furry Frederick's of Hollywood getup that would embarrass Mrs. Roper during Amok time? Or with sex toys, joy buzzers, vibrating whatzits, and all that? Don't get me started. Coals to Newcastle, my friend. I've got sex toys coming out your ass. [http://www.babeland.com]

Am I leaving anything out? Absolutely. So many manners to mind. Oh, but I'll hit you with more stuff in the future—know that. Meanwhile, thank you, come again, and please don't ask me for my home phone number. That is, not unless you're planning to give me your mother's in return.

SONGS OF SADISM

In S&M, atmosphere is everything. But of all the elements a mistress combines to set the tone for her session—lighting, costume, implements of destruction—there's one that so often seems woefully neglected. And that is music.

It's really unfortunate, because choosing a sound track for your session ought to be one of the more enjoyable decisions a mistress makes during her day. The music you choose to whip by can make or break a mood. Yet so often, I see mistresses leaving this crucial creative decision to chance.

First, music serves a practical function. Namely, sessions get loud. A hard mega bass does wonders to drown out the ass-thwacking being delivered to the client in the adjoining dungeon. Sure, you might have a slave who gets off on the voyeuristic thrill of hearing his subbie brethren's sessions, but sometimes the tone of one kills the other. The slave in Dungeon #2 is a brooding, bleeding, burning human sacrifice for the mistress he adores; meanwhile, the guy in #3 is a miniature schnauzer. See what I'm saying? Plaid and paisley just don't mix.

Also, when you're in session, music drowns out the sound of your fellow mistresses shuffling about the premises. You really don't want your slave overhearing your coworkers' watercooler shop talk. Dominas nattering on about errant boyfriends, yeast infections (latex is a bitch), and overdue term papers can be a real mystique shatterer.

And mistresses do, on occasion, discuss the particulars of their sessions with one another and can be mercilessly candid. While it's generally considered bad form to whip and tell, we're human, and sometimes we need the reality check of saying, "Oh my God, guys—you'll never believe what this guy can do with three surgical gloves and a tweezer!" Sometimes, a loud Tom Waits tape is the only thing standing between you and your client realizing he might be next up for dissection. Privacy, please!

Here's a phenomenon I've witnessed time and again, and it never fails to needle me: the thoughtless abuse of the musical component. It's not only bad mistressing; it's bad business.

Today, Mistress X is having a session with Orville, a genteel old fart who likes to get his neck scissored between the calves of a woman wearing an olde-tyme saloon girl stockings-and-garters getup. He's also into being whipped with a heavy cane, which practically broadcasts the fact that he once did time in an all-boys boarding school in either Europe or Canada.

Now, Mistress X drags Orville into the dungeon by his ear, being careful not to dislodge his hearing aid. She cues up a CD and prepares to cane his old ass like a cheap flea-market rattan love seat. The music begins to swell . . . a crescendo of barnyard rutting . . . and it's the musical stylings of a band named Der Klüsterfuck or some similar nonsense.

And I'm thinking, *Jesus on a pony*. Not because it's one of those especially hip bands with seven fans in six countries (surely you know the kind) but because Orville is probably not one of them. In fact he was born in that period of time when World War I was commonly referred to as the Great War and he thinks that Courtney Love has something to do with knights, nobility, and maidens named

Marian. This is one of life's few moments when you are allowed to hope that someone is deaf as a post.

I'm here to tell you that a mutually agreeable musical selection is your basic session right, be you mistress or slave. Especially in the world of commercial S&M, where a person is paying to enact a specific fantasy. It's that important; I just don't think a client should be subjected to music he hates any more than he should be forced to endure cigarette smoke or body odor or bad tattoos. Unless it's a clearly stated part of the torture; a different matter entirely.

You should discuss the sound track at the same time that you would consult with your slave on any other session basics, like clothing and whether or not you can leave marks. Don't be surprised if he says he doesn't care for any kind of musical accompaniment at all; just the dulcet tones of your sweet little voice will do, Mistress Sirena. In which case, you will make him sing for you. (I'll tell you about that session sometime.)

Unless you enjoy dragging your entire cassette collection to work with you (or if you have a slave to do the dragging), you're going to need to streamline your aural kit down to the basics. And make sure it's all stuff that you like—you're going to let your slave make his "choice" from the five or six selections that you have mandated.

Let me upend my own black knapsack and see what falls out.

First up, and my personal favorite, the oldies mix tape. Yes, I said oldies. Torch songs, twists, and oddities from the 1950s and '60s. Why? Because it's some of the only music, radiowise, that I can stomach. I absolutely refuse to keep in step with the parade of crap that's out there these days, that stinking compost heap turned over regularly by sterile old bean counters in their corporate silos. I'd rather listen to the crap from my parents' era. At least it's finite.

And it's more than just wallpaper—it's powerful Memory Lane pavement. Dion, the Platters, anything produced by Phil Spector, and so on, that's the music that was playing at the time in his life he remembers most fondly—the bud of his virile youth.

But I suppose you're wondering why I would want my slave to feel good, much less virile, given the context of our encounter. As

I've said, the musical underpinning is basic. I like my slaves to feel comfortable when they're being tormented—no accidental discomfort to distract them from the deliberate discomfort that I am inflicting. So if I'm going to tear the man down, brick by testosterone-soaked brick, I want to set my starting point somewhere close to his personal best. It just makes for better drama.

Plus, just you listen to those oldie lyrics in the context of whips and chains and hot wax and nipple clamps—they take on a dazzling, sinister subtext. Dig back even further, to all that quavery 1920s and '30s stuff, and you won't have to wonder whether or not they knew about that thing we call B&D. *Is it love that binds me helpless to your heart?*

I've got a jazz tape and a classical tape in here: Mingus's *Black Saint and the Sinner Lady,* which everyone should own; but the name on the classical I can't quite make out. Rachmaninoff, I think. Truthfully, I keep it only as a kind of default setting, in case Slave Boy and I can't come up with anything else we both can tolerate. You can't go wrong with classical, as long as it wasn't recorded by, say, the Toms River Chamber Orchestra and Hibachi Club.

Now here's the real deal, Pallie, some of the ol' Francis Albert Sinatra. A musical food group all his own. *The Reprise Recordings* contains all the standards, of course, and I've got one live tape from Paris, 1962, where he's in rare form. Sauced. For some reason, leg and foot fetishists seem to love Sinatra the most. I think it's because Frank trips them back to that pre-p.c. era, when a fella could admire a nice set of stems without a dame suing him for sexual harassment. Sinatra and S&M, perfect together. [http://www.accessplace.com/sinatra.htm]

And last, my favorite tape, "Town Without Pity"—the Gene Pitney classic. (Don't even think of substituting the modern-day Brian Setzer cover; a noble effort, but hardly the same.) You *know* you know the song, an over-the-top epic of cruel fates conspiring against star-crossed teenagers in a society that just doesn't understand. For those of us who engage in clandestine rites of sadomasochism, we feel your pain, Loverboy. The poor yearning sap sings the shit out of this song; you can just see him crumpling to his knees and appealing to an uncaring sky. I've got a tape of "Town Without Pity" playing over and over on a ninety-minute Maxell; this gives us about twenty-five rounds of poignant, repetitious heartache.

Sometimes, I'll use this tape for a session. I don't consult with my slave on this particular selection, either. Because in this town, I'm the sheriff. I'm also the judge, jury, and disc jockey. Who knows, maybe you'll get tired of hearing the song. But I never do. As a matter of fact, you'll never guess what I'm listening to right now.

A VERY CROSS DRESSER

The world of professional mistressing, like so many areas of life, is a place where many people are capable of being passably good, but only a rare few have what it takes to be truly great. Someday you may have the chops to do dominance in lederhosen and a root-beer barrel, who knows? But until that day, the astute neophyte knows she'd better dress the part.

In any freelance enterprise, you've got to spend money to make money. That's why I always tell new mistresses not to wait until they've scored their first session to buy themselves the proper gear. They may find themselves waiting a very long time.

A good outfit serves a dual function. First is the perception-becomes-reality factor. In the dungeon, a client may think of me—the nonmistress me, that is—whatever way he likes: as a slacker, an enterprising college student, single mother on the make, and so on. His very presence, however, indicates a willingness to play along. He *wants* to accept me as a sadistic hellion of a bitch interested solely in his degradation and forced servitude. Who am I to disappoint? The shiny, forbidding fetish gear is what helps me to walk, talk, and act the part—just you try spreading joy in six-inch pumps and a nineteen-inch corset. For the novice mistress, or one who isn't naturally predisposed to bad behavior, the evil armor is guaranteed to help.

The second function is the fetish factor. There are some very sincere fetishists out there whose session depends on a lick of a sweat-soaked leather boot, the scent of a latex corset, or the corkscrewing back seam of a pair of flesh-colored, reinforced-heel, thigh-high stockings. Beyond that, there are some clients who do engage in S&M play at home; what makes sneaking out to their local dungeon a special treat is seeing all the made-up dominas in their magnificent showgirl attire. Decked out, the intractable male ego presumes, for them and only them.

Then, of course, there are certain asshole clients—guys who'd be penny-ante dickheads no matter where you found them—who get off solely on the power trip of making the mistress change her outfit, just because they know they can request that. They're likely the same guys who get wood watching the service-station attendant hustle to check their oil even when they know they put in a fresh quart that morning.

So let's suppose you're new to our dungeon, and you've somehow secured Mistress Ruby as your official S&M style consultant. Here's what I'd put together for your trousseau. We'll start with the basics.

In S&M, *basics* means leather, and lots of it. But the wrong leather marks you as a cliché—an HBO *Real Sex* extra. Wrong leather is cheap leather, a menopausal housewife's attempt to spice up her marriage. If you can purchase it in a mall, it's not the real deal. Ditto for anything fringed.

I'm sure you can get off the bus at the Port Authority and find a nice black skirt in your price range at Teepee Town. And I'm sure you think you can snip off the powwow fringe without your coworkers catching wise. But you will always know in your heart that it came with a headdress and a bolo tie, and that knowledge will banish it to the back of your locker forevermore, Kemosabe.

Good leather is a classic. It's thick and double-stitched with lots of shiny buckles and snaps and zippers to distract your slave from whatever punishment you happen to be preparing. And it shouldn't have more lining to it than leather—it's the one fabric you really want to feel against your skin. Why should your slaves have all the fun? If you're savvy, you'll buy items you can wear with your lay clothes; this will ease the pain of parting with $150 for, say, a vest.

But before we continue, here's the most important advice of all. With few exceptions, you should always buy the best. And don't walk out of any store with your second choice of anything, especially if it's merely in the name of saving money. If you're already spending a couple hundred bucks, another fifty, another hundred won't matter. Trust me, you will have absorbed the difference long before you learn to love your almost-perfect purchase. Its very existence will remind you that you just didn't think you were worthy of having what you want—in clothing, and in life. And there's very little good that can come of that. This goes for all things, not just mistressing.

But back to the fashion show. Next there's PVC, polyvinyl chloride—think Catwoman's catsuit in *Batman Returns.* Personally, I'm not a big fan of the stuff since it's gone so mainstream. To me, it doesn't so much say mistress as anorexic model/club kid. But the prices have come down, and you should consider it wardrobe filler. But be warned: When it rips there's not a damned thing you can do about it. Don't even *think* of trying to "solder" it back together with a bent wire hanger that you've heated with a Zippo (not that I've tried, of course).

Then there's latex, a personal favorite. It's hot, in more ways than one. If you've ever wondered how many quarts of liquid a body excretes in an hour, just don a latex shirt and you will have your answer. Most good latex is lined, pulling moisture away from the skin. But even with the lining, do yourself a favor and don't buy latex pants or shorts, unless they happen to come with a year's supply of Monistat 7. If not, prepare to bake bread in your trousers.

Now you'll need stockings; the more and varied the better. Take a trip to Lee's Mardi Gras, the transvestite/cross-dresser store in the meatpacking district, and load up the shopping cart. You'll want the classic fishnet, the thigh-high, in both black and flesh tone, freestanding and with garter belt.

Most of all, you'll want anything with a back seam, and any style that seems to have been discontinued around the time of the Kennedy assassination. Those were the years when most clients were coming of age; these were the stockings their original objects of desire were wearing when those fetishes began to form. While you're at it, buy yourself a set of falsies. Jane Russell, Jayne Mansfield, Marilyn Monroe—"big" stars of that same era.

Shoes must be high, arched, and scary. Of your first two pairs, one should have a closed toe, the other open. Ankle straps are a plus. With the right shoes, you will no doubt attract foot fetishists. And those foot fetishists will invariably purchase you shoes, and then those shoes will be the ones you wear. Say whatever you like about a man with a fetish, but he knows what he likes. You'll always make money in his shoes.

Two other items for your starter kit: first, you'll need a nice-but-not-too-nice dress. It can be either black or red—doesn't matter—but it must be figure-forgiving. This is the dress you will wear when it's that feminine time and you feel simply wretched but must report to the dungeon anyway, because you used up your cramp excuse last week, when for no good reason you didn't feel like working. This should be an over-the-head, quick-change garment you can spice up with gloves and/or studded choker; it will serve you well in a host of other emergencies.

Finally, there's the coverall, slippers and a robe or muumuu, something you can throw on to safely answer the door for food deliveries. Do you really want to be masturbation fodder for the Chicken Delight delivery boy?

When you get to be as jaded and accustomed as I, you may want to mix things up a bit. And, over time, you're bound to accumulate some very specific accessories (a sheriff's badge, a pince-nez, and so on). Eventually, you'll have put together some costumes for yourself. Here's a rundown of the many faces of Ruby:

Evil Bitch Boss: Maybe it has something to do with my aversion to gainful employment, but somehow I find it so satisfying to act out the horrors of the workplace. I've got this really sharp, tight, gray flannel suit, the skirt slit way up high. It does double duty for Sadistic Governess scenes. See me attired thusly, and clients almost always want to get spanked. "Find me that memo, peon, or your ass is mine!"

Naughty Schoolgirl: The genuine plaid-pleated article; so glad I didn't burn it upon graduation. The older the client, the more effective the costume. Clients like to be caught masturbating in the teachers lounge in this number.

The Doctor Is In(sane): I've got a white lab coat, complete with phony bloodstains, white stockings, and white pumps. Oh, plus a strap-on underneath. "Dr. Ruby, my dick hurts." "Really? Does it hurt when I go like *this* . . . ?"

Tomboy Boy Scout: "I promise to be honest, helpful, courteous, brave . . . and to kick the living shit out of any kid who thinks I can't make a lanyard." I beat up my fellow scouts at every opportunity. Clients who go for this look tend to be Female Supremacists or latent homosexuals.

There's tons of other gack in my closet—Geisha Girl, Society Whore, Paranoid Militia Member, Aerobics Instructor with a Heart of Titanium. Unless a client specifically requests it, I'm loath to trot any of it out. The truth is, the greatest enjoyment I derive from my fetish wardrobe is when I wear it around my own house. At work, I've got the chops—I don't need to rely on the pomp and pageantry. So what do I wear for my sessions? Lederhosen and a root-beer barrel, of course.

MONEY MATTERS

Unless otherwise noted, all monies are divided fifty-fifty between the mistress and the house.

- Half-hour session: $100
- One hour: $180
- Two hours: $320
- Multiple-hour sessions: discounted at the discretion of the management
- Two-mistress special: $270 (three-way split among mistresses and house)

In times of poverty, any of the above can be negotiated.

By now you may have noticed what seems to be a cruel paradox: scads of money floating around; consistently impoverished mistresses.

There are reasons for this—some practical, some esoteric.

Work Ethic

For most people, making $600 in a single shift would be a terrific incentive to cash in by working as many days as possible. Mistresses, however, do not share this opinion. A banner day is usually taken as a signal to call in sick until you are broke again.

Also, not every day bears fruit. That $600 you made in an afternoon? Did I mention that you had to endure four days of nothing before that afternoon happened?

Outside Influences

Drug addiction, mooching boyfriends, mooching drug-addict boyfriends; expensive taste in footwear. Need I say more?

Dollars and Senselessness

Unlike the exploited proletariat, we are not estranged from the fruits of our labor—we are estranged from the *labor* of our labor. Money tends to lose its meaning, its worth, when you make so much so easily. Granted, that's the feature that attracted us to this brand of employment. But at the same time, with no apparent relationship between effort and reward, it's easy to apply this standard—or lack thereof—to your spending habits as well.

Don't forget that many of your clients made their fortunes in a similar manner—in the stock market, through consulting, even white-collar crime. Why do you think they're so willing to blow it in a dungeon? Somehow, the money they made on those slippery slopes of illegality has a way of slithering through your French-manicured fingers as well.

There was a time when I practiced my own brand of tithing, almost to the point of superstition. I used to need to blow, like, 5 to 10 percent of the day's take on my way home, as if I thought something bad would happen if I didn't.

But what's telling is the stuff I'd purchase—nothing expensive, such as jewelry, but something completely ordinary, yet ridiculously priced. Like one of those seven-dollar plums from Balducci's, or a forty-dollar jar of mineral mask. Now I understand what I was *really* doing—not pampering myself with fancy fruit or designer mud, but paying homage to the absurdity of money itself.

SELLING THE (PSYCHO) DRAMA

Who can forget how O.J.'s infamous freeway chase sent white Ford Broncos (bloodstains not included) sailing out of the showrooms? Conversely, the cattle industry took a nosedive after Oprah's segment on Mad Cow Disease. And a few summers back, that Smashing Pumpkins keyboardist OD'd on a brand of heroin called Redrum; the corpse wasn't even cold and junkies all over New York City were scrambling to score the killer smack.

Every industry—from the blackest black market to the most tight-assed bureaucracy—waxes and wanes according to external influences. The world of commercial S&M is no exception. But considering the nature of our commodity, the factors that determine the boom or bust of spanking sales are far more fickle, more tenuous. They exist not just in the headlines and the NASDAQ, but within the deepest recesses of the psyche.

Today, I'm not even going to hazard my usual guess as to what kind of psychological road map propels a man to move from the womb and into his oedipal phase, take a sharp left at adolescence, give up blow jobs for the E.R.A. in college, power-tie into his thirties, pop a wheelie through his midlife crisis, and then *wham!* slide into a pair of Pampers for his secret other life as Mr. I. P. Didie, the Adult Baby.

Because that's not even the weirdest part of the phenomenon. Once the psychic stage is set, what then gives him the idea that today is *the* day to cancel his meetings, lie to Mrs. Didie, and cab it uptown to see me? *It's time to make piddle in my poodie; please hold all my calls.*

And then what makes *three* of these guys—Adult Babies, that is—decide to show up at our dungeon in a single afternoon? It does work in cycles like that, you know. Is it merely coincidence? Zeitgeist? Something in the water supply? Something on TV? I'd really like to see what the market researchers have to say about *that* one.

Of course, wherever there are trends, there are people trying to predict those trends. In our case, it's more than just recreational speculation; this is our bread and butter here (some days, more like bread and water). On any given shift, dominas will roll into the dungeon sipping coffee, bitching about our boyfriends/girlfriends, and so on. And, guaranteed, pooling our resources to prognosticate how much human traffic we're going to see that evening.

A typical watercooler conversation might go like this: "Supposed to rain hard tonight." Translation: good for business.

"Yeah, but it's the last payday of the month." Bad, very bad.

"But Monday was a holiday—we're gonna get all the guys that couldn't come in then." This could go either way.

"I don't know, I'm feeling a green aura around this place."

Optimism prevails—auras being as reliable as anything else—and we all go back to drawing on our eyebrows. But then Carlos, our hulking Samoan security guy, comes huffing into the lounge and asks if he may briefly commandeer the TV. "Playoffs tonight," he explains.

And that's when all the good feeling drains from us and we resign ourselves to a night of catching up on our needlepoint. Because for that moment, we know exactly how a stripper feels when she shakes her moneymaker at a guy who's ignoring her ass crack in favor of the TV monitor above the bar: sporting events induce a hard-on all their own.

Admittedly, there's very little, apart from advertising in the fetish papers and brushing up on her phone manner, that a mistress can do to compel clients to come in for a session. Yet our financial well-being does depend on knowing what kind of business to expect, one week to the next, so that we can budget ourselves accordingly. We are, after all, freelancers, contracted laborers, if you will. It's feast or famine, and we're flying through the air without a net; no job security, no dental plan.

Take Presidents' Day, for instance. A great day for business, because although most people have the day off, it's a holiday with very little emotional resonance. Even the most sentimental girlfriend does not really expect to celebrate the births of George and Abe with her man. In fact it affords a client a near-perfect alibi, to dash out for a couple of hours, maybe catch up on some "work" at the "office."

So in the spirit of the holiday, you may have cabbed home with your pocketbook stuffed full of your own dead presidents. But before you go dashing out to buy yourself that cunning little PVC ensemble, you've got to consider whether or not that's your money for the week, or if you'd be wise to make it last through Passover, a season when mistresses also ask God to deliver us from the land of bondage.

In order to stay afloat, we guess and then second-guess; we look at the stats from this day last year; we consult with the Weather Channel and scan the headlines and schedule our vacations accordingly. We become equal parts Nostradamus, Al Roker, and the conspiracy kook down the street. When all else proves inconclusive, we may peruse the horoscopes.

What results is a handicapping system that would make Jimmy the Greek look like a simpleton. If I had the computer know-how, I'd invent a program that would take into account all the factors that make business good or bad. In the morning, a mistress could plug in all the variables and decide what she ought to bring to work that day: her comfiest pair of killing boots, a trashy John Grisham novel, or her homework from school.

Here's a list—and it's by no means complete—of conditions that affect our industry, either directly or indirectly: weather, sporting events, religious holidays, regular holidays, state of the stock market, time of year, time of month, time of day, tax season, the unemployment rate, current events, parades and festivals, alternate-side-of-the-street parking rules suspended/enforced, police crackdowns, papal visits, epidemics and health scares, and, of course, what's on television.

Let's take a look at some of the biggies. Weather tops our list. From what I've seen, a little precipitation is a good thing. When the sky is blue and clouds are high and puffy, few men would elect to spend lunchtime in a dank, windowless bunker of a dungeon. And this has more to do with scoping skirts than soaking up the sun—especially on those first spring-awakening days when ties are loosened, jackets abandoned, and people start venturing out of the mole holes they've been stuck in, white-skinned and sexless, all winter.

On the other hand, too much precipitation is bad—no one likes to brave a blizzard only to be told to strip naked and sit on a cold stone floor. (A tip for the frugal fetishist: some of the better dungeons are hip to these trends, and will offer discounted session rates during extraordinarily beautiful or inclement weather.)

Show me a room full of dominas, and I will show you a group of women as familiar with the Dow Jones Industrial Average as any of their Wall Street slaves. Since so many of our clients play the market, a bull or bear day usually applies to our trading floor as well.

Then there are the darkest days of all. That's right, religious holidays. Two words: Forget it. Don't even bother coming to work, and this goes triple for Jewish holidays. In fact, you'll never realize how much of your clientele is composed of nice Jewish men until you work a Yom Kippur and keep checking to make sure the ringer on the phone isn't broken.

But I'd like to take this opportunity to reassure all the clients' wives (and don't think I'm not talking to *you*) that no matter what human depravities your husband has been enjoying—if he's been spat upon, trussed like a turkey, or worse—he is always extremely conscientious about getting home to you in time for sundown/ mosque/5:30 mass. So please don't be *too* upset when you discover he's spent your birthday money on a custom-made Sissymaid outfit for his Friday afternoon sessions with me. He's actually very devout, you know.

As for the other factors I've cited, current events seem to provide the most satisfying cause-and-effect chain. For instance, do you remember when that guy got into trouble for stealing Marla Maples's shoes? Yep, you guessed it, foot sessions increased. I remember one shoe enthusiast who even wanted to act out the moment of truth: *"What do you think you're doing?! Get your face out of my Manolo Blahniks and sniff my sling-backs, or I'm calling the Donald!"*

Just in case you think you're getting the hang of dungeon odds-making, I've got to warn you, just as in science class, for each action there is an equal and opposite reaction. Here's where you get to use your powers of counterintuition.

Take Valentine's Day, usually bad for business. That's because it's a day associated with relationships, love, and other forms of cavity-inducing sweetness. But for every Romeo enjoying a dip in a champagne glass–shaped Jacuzzi with his paramour, there's another poor schmuck who's just had his heart ripped out through his asshole by some ungrateful bitch who doesn't want anything more to do with him. So where does Disappointment Boy go for consolation? That's exactly right.

I know what you're thinking. You're thinking that there's no real way to handicap dungeon business. Too many conflicting variables, too many uncertainties. And you'd be right. But I've got one last trick up my sleeve—an oddsmaking law that is just about foolproof.

It's the law that says that the day your feet are ripped to hamburger, you will get foot-fetish clients. If you're menstruating, a water-sports client will offer you $800 for a cup of your pee—full-bodied burgundy, however, is the only deal-breaker; that grosses him out.

If you come to work with the Hong Kong flu, you will be required to jump around the dungeon like a cheerleader in the bloom of health. The day that you're well but call in sick anyway, because it's Rosh Hashanah and you don't want to waste your time, your home phone keeps ringing and ringing. Finally answer it in your best phony deathbed voice: "Uuuhlo?"

And it's the dungeon owner, who says it's a good thing you're sick or else she'd kill you, a client just left the building with $10,000, cash, in his pocket, which he had wanted to spend on you and only you, and he had specifically come in on the holiday because he figured it wouldn't be so busy. And you've just missed out. But that's no dungeon law, that's Murphy's Law, and it applies just as well to any business—greed-based, charity, or otherwise—on the planet.

THE OMEGA MISTRESS

There's this dream—actually, more like a nightmare—that I have from time to time. I call it the Omega Man. I step out of the subway and into a city from which all humanity has been completely erased. In this abandoned Manhattan, alternate-side-of-the-street parking has not only been suspended, it has been forgotten. Cars, buses, and taxis—all locked, all deserted—choke the intersections in an eternal traffic jam.

The delis are dark, but the flowers are fresh; the curtains are drawn in every apartment window. It's so quiet, I can hear the traffic lights change up and down Sixth Avenue. I cover my ears and run and run and keep on running. Eventually I realize where I'm going: the dungeon. I ring the bell and hold my breath. Finally, someone buzzes me in. Turns out it's not the Apocalypse after all; it's just Christmas Day in New York City. And I have to report to work.

There's a basic rule of dungeon economics that even the neophyte mistress understands: during the holidays, business is dead. As far as Christmas is concerned, expect to make your money in the rush that precedes it. Clients out stimulating the economy usually have no problem blowing a couple hundred bucks gifting themselves. And doing Santa's work makes a great cover story for the wife and kids. As long as you return home with a surprise or two—something other than a red, welted ass, that is—no one's gonna ask where you've been.

But as for the joyous day itself—forget about coming to work. And I'm not just talking Christmas here; I'm talking Thanksgiving, Easter, Yom Kippur, New Year's, and Rosh Hashanah, plus all of Passover and all of Chanukah. These are the hallowed days of home and family, and most clients understand that as the rule.

But just as every rule has its exception, sometimes, in the dungeon, these days do extraordinary business. Basically, if you put out some milk and cookies, if you don your gayest fetish gear—hell, if you so much as turn on the phone—clients will come dashing down your chimney.

Given the lifestyles that many mistresses tend to embrace, it's easy to see why some would consider spending the holidays at work. Some of them just don't do the Judeo-Christian thing—some are Wiccans, atheists, disciples of Zoroaster, you name it. Some come from out of town and just can't make it home; still others would like to see the day come and go without undue fanfare.

And the fact is, we make a pretty merry time of it. Just like you and yours, we eat and we drink, maybe exchange some presents. We pile onto the boss's bed and order pay-per-view, maybe some Ultimate Fighting, maybe some pornography. If the business phone rings, it rings; often, by the time it does, we're so busy yakking and eating and grappling for the remote that for a moment we forget what we're doing here. Really, it's the only day of the year that making money is beside the point.

Me, I grew up around here; I've already got a pack of relatives that expect my attendance at the holiday dinner table. Celebrating the season with my *other* dysfunctional family isn't the only reason you'll find me in an S&M parlor on Christmas afternoon or New Year's Eve.

Truth be told, I do it for the clients. Not because I can't stand to see the fetishists of America go unattended for a day—if I wanted to feel benevolent, I'd give my time to a soup kitchen. Nor do I do it for the money; this time of year, a day's income makes little difference either way.

No, I do it for the weirdness of it all, the perversity—that, and for the insight you can glean only from doing one thing when the rest of the world is doing almost exactly the opposite.

Let's take Christmas. A guy who calls a dungeon on December 25 is a client you are unlikely to see any other day of the year. It's almost as if he's been invented specially for the occasion; and for that, he comes with his own unique characteristics. He's either got way too much money, and tips like crazy, or not enough, and we cut him a break. He's absolutely staggered when we answer the phone. And unlike your everyday client, this guy almost always keeps his appointment, often calling several times prior, as if to make sure he hasn't dreamt us up in the first place.

The sessions are remarkable only in that they tend toward corporal tortures—flogging, whipping, and so on—and rarely toward role play or heavy psychological scenes. They're seeking a kind of gratification and release that doesn't demand deep thinking. Most of these guys take multiple-hour sessions, and for most of that time, the guy's explaining exactly how he came to be in a dungeon on Christmas Day. These guys *always* have a story.

And on this day, we get to hear them all. The businessman from Omaha who's stuck in the big city, wants to act crazy, wants to get wild, wants to do something quintessentially New York. Most of all, he wants to be somewhere that won't remind him of the warm meal he's missing back home. The cable-TV producer who thought he'd check out the scene—purely for the purposes of "research," he'll tell us—on a day he figured we wouldn't be too busy. He ends up staying eight, ten hours, suspended upside down in full rigging. A mighty sophisticated request for a first-time client, and it's hard to do research when you're blindfolded and gagged.

These are not so much stories as excuses. It's as if he needs to make his alibi to *us* rather than to the people he allegedly left behind at the Christmas tree or the menorah candles or the Easter basket or turkey dinner.

But you needn't file your explanations with me. I know the long and illustrious history of lonely men seeking comfort on the shoulders of strippers and prostitutes—and bartenders and cabbies and mistresses, too. Because we're paid, and because we're here, there's this perception that we're lonely and disenfranchised too, and that's what enables him to reveal himself to us on a day when his shrink is out of town with his family.

The so-called holiday blues get a really bad rap in this country, where perfection and happiness are a perpetually sparkling toilet bowl and tortilla chips that never lose their crunch. But a deep and full-bodied sadness is actually as necessary a part of the season as the joy we're supposed to be celebrating. Think about it: there's no room at the inn for the pregnant mother; the Jews are kicked out of their homeland; poor Rudolph can't join in any reindeer games; George Bailey wants to jump off a bridge. Without the pain of exile, there can be no ecstasy of redemption.

Sometimes I'll sit out a holiday simply because I'm sick of all the obligations and manufactured good cheer; tuning in to my own loneliness becomes the only way I can appreciate making contact with other people. Take a walk through Midtown on Christmas morning and you'll notice there's not much difference between holidays in the city and a natural disaster—earthquake, flood, and yes, even nuclear annihilation.

Nothing's quite the way you're used to, and so the normal codes of conduct are suspended. You walk right down the middle of the street a little ways; a bum turns from his piss and gives you a rose. By the time you get to where you're going, not only are you glad to be received, you experience a rare camaraderie that's a lot like that of castaways sitting out a nasty storm.

I remember this one client who came to see us on Christmas afternoon. Jolly and squat, you might have taken him for St. Nick himself, except that he was as hairless as an egg and half-Filipino. The little guy ran us ragged, exhausting three different mistresses with six hours of sound spanking. He tipped like crazy and never stopped grinning—even when, at his request, we literally lit his ass on fire.

So infectious was his cheer that eventually we invited him into the back for a cup of nog, some pie, and a few rounds of pornography. He was a real asset to the party, able to spot a C-section scar at fifteen paces, mixing up a batch of "recipe" in the sink that got us thoroughly hammered. At one point, he leapt atop the punishment horse and began riffing on *A Christmas Carol* with a passion that I think surprised even him: *Are there no titty bars? No peep shows? No whorehouses, operating in full vigor?*

Then he told us he had a surprise for us: turns out his wife and stepkids had abandoned him that morning for real and for good, leaving no more than a note and a stack of unopened presents—his and theirs—beneath the tree. If he wanted to step out for an hour or so, would we still be here when he returned?

Now, if this were a TV movie or a news report, you'd expect the guy to go home and swallow a gun or something. But this being a true story, the dungeon scored a humidifier and a spice rack; one mistress got a remote-control race car. Our new friend took great mirth in presenting the dungeon owner with a silver-plated stopwatch, courtesy of his soon-to-be ex-wife.

Me, I got a sweater, which was the wrong color and didn't really fit, but no matter. We were just happy to welcome him back into the fold. Never doubted for a second he'd return. After all, we were the last, the best, and the only party in town.

THE BEARDED LADY

It's unfortunate, but not everybody will celebrate your S&M career. These people may include loved ones, landlords, and the terminally unenlightened. Sure, *you* might know that your job does not involve sex or illegality, or that you're only doing it to fund your independent film, or that you're planning to ditch it for grad school next fall. But trust me, not everyone will choose to take the long view of things. To avoid unnecessary strife—for you *and* them—you will need to know how to conceal your profession.

1. The Career Canard: This is the thing that you say you do in order to alibi all those hours you spend flogging businessmen. For practical reasons, this should be a gig with flexible hours, a vague location, and absolutely no number at which you can be reached. Telemarketing and catering are ideal, ditto flyer distribution and dog-walking.

   Nowadays, the Internet offers limitless opportunities for nonspecific employment: website design, network interface management, hypertext consulting. I made up those last ones; you, too, should feel free to get creative—the field is wide open! These work especially well with computer-challenged oldsters. But be warned: Only techie-beard if you really know your bits and bauds. When Aunt Nellie's screen hangs up, she'll be expecting you to make a house call.

2. Asset Management: You must treat your cash, when you have it, like it's the spoils of a bank robbery or kidnapping. In other words, don't make any big purchases. Become a beard-conscious shopper—as a $12.50-an-hour "temp," can you really afford those Manolos?

   Of course I'm not saying you can't treat yourself; you work hard, sort of, for your money. You've just got to be careful not to parade too much wealth around the people you're trying to mislead. There are only so many times a person can win the Pick-3 or receive a thoughtful gift from a well-to-do friend. Too many pricey trinkets, and even the most naive relative will begin to suspect you're a call girl.

3. The Art of the Lie: Maybe you're as slick as snot on a doorknob. If so, you don't need my help. But even if you're a lousy liar, don't despair; you can use your honest reputation to your advantage. You see, in order to be a good liar, it helps if people already think you're a *bad* liar. Meanwhile, when no one's looking, you're going to have to brush up on your technique.

   First, keep your lies simple. Offering too much information makes you sound dodgy and eager to please—or worse, eager to be believed. At the same time, you'll want to drop one or two specific details. Never say, "I'm catering this weekend," when you can say, "I'm catering an *outdoor wedding* this weekend." See the difference?

   Rehearse your fib on someone who doesn't matter before you have to lay it on someone who does. You'll find that the repetition will help you internalize the details, and this will smoothe out any hitches or stammers. Remember, it's not a lie if *you* believe it.

   Most important, realize that it's terribly arrogant to presume that your double life is any more scandalous than anyone else's. Console yourself with the knowledge that everybody's life is weirder than it appears to be. You're a dominatrix—of all people, you should understand that.

Unfortunately, all the pep talks didn't prepare me for the time that my two lives nearly crashed into each other. On paper, my beard theory worked just fine; when things hit close to home, however, it failed to address how I'd actually feel.

MY LIFE AS A DOG

I'm here to tell you, having a double life ain't all it's cracked up to be. Sure, from the outside, it might *seem* romantic—kind of like having two lovers fighting over you—but ultimately, it just left me feeling queasy, with a constant sense of impending doom. You're always waiting for the day when the lies won't add up, when a single careless remark trips the wires of suspicion and one set of whereabouts fails to cover the other. That's your personal Armageddon, my friend, the day your worlds finally collide. And then you've got an awful lot of explaining to do.

As a dominatrix, I'm no stranger to double—and even triple—identities, to duality and deception. To my clients, I'm a ball-busting sadist, an evil baby-sitter, the patron saint of cross-dressers—depends on what's paying the rent that day. In the publishing world, I'm a writer ass-deep in scholarly S&M research. To my parents, I'm a dutiful daughter and semistarving artist—an artist with a penchant for expensive leather coats and luxury vacations, but starving nonetheless. And to the schoolchildren of three counties—pre-K to fourth grade—I am Barkley, the Smart Dog.

My relationship with Barkley began about a year and a half into my dungeon career. Ah, but those were the salad days of S&M, and I remember them with the misty-eyed reverence most baby boomers reserve for the sixties. The market hadn't yet become completely oversaturated with strippers trying to cash in on this latest adult-entertainment craze, and so for those of us who'd come aboard early on, the field was wide open.

Like most pioneers, we thought it would last forever, which of course it didn't. But for a while there, never have so few made so much doing so little.

With the money, however, came certain problems. I soon realized that in order to conceal my newfound identity, I would also have to conceal my newfound wealth. Naturally, I knew better than to show up at family functions in leather corsets and killing boots; the trick was not to show up in Versace.

I swallowed my pride and maintained the slacker-daughter look they'd come to love and accept. All the spoils of a successful mistress career—the stereo, the appliances, the $500 electric unit with the scrotal-shock attachment—stayed locked away in my apartment, safe from the curious eyes of my nearest and dearest.

Then one day, as they say, the ax just fell. My Sicilian grandmother, sweet and shrewd old lady that she was, had always taken a critical interest in my career; more specifically, the fact that I *had* no career. As far as she could tell, being a writer was employment at its vaguest—no hours? no commute? no health insurance?—and she'd made it quite clear she'd be happier if I worked in the circus.

But now she had cancer, and it was terminal; facing the end of her life, she'd made peace with the fact that whatever I wanted to do with mine was fine by her. To confer her blessing, she was going to pay the rent on my apartment until the day she died or until I came to my senses and got a *real* job. Somehow I knew that being a dominatrix wasn't exactly what she had in mind.

I was horrified. The notion of my dying grandmother forking over her last few Social Security checks to pay for an apartment that housed, among other things, a scrotal-shock unit and a mattress full

of money—money I'd made beating the piss out of degenerates—
was a prospect more perverse than anything I'd ever encountered in
the underworld. Painful as it was, there was only one thing to do: I'd
have to get a job—a visible job, with a visible paycheck—and fast.
That's when Barkley the Smart Dog came to the rescue. My
mother, who was a teacher, knew another teacher who knew a
school-board administrator who was looking for someone to do
these inspirational "presentations" in the public schools a couple of
mornings a week.

It sounded like the perfect job for me. After all, didn't I know that
it was cool to stay in school and that hugs were better than drugs?
The hours, too, were ideal. I'd be done with the kiddies in plenty of
time to make my 12:30 booking with, say, Diaper David or Philip
the Ass Guy.

I showed up for my first assembly, full of piss and vinegar and
bullshit missionary zeal. Backstage, I met with Wanda, the program
coordinator, a surprisingly hip old lady with dual hearing aids
who'd probably been traveling the Barkley circuit when *Don't* Tune
In, Turn On, or Drop Out had been its mantra.

She gave me the Barkley drill: First the presentation, which would
distill all the wisdom that modern-day bumper-sticker sloganeering
had to offer. Then, a short "rap session" where the children would
voice their questions and concerns. Finally, Barkley, that lovable
mutt, would emerge from behind the curtains, do his little dance,
shake his furry rump, and rain crayons and coloring books upon the
masses.

I told Wanda that I hadn't exactly planned a speech. But if it was
all right with her, I would be more than happy to share with the students the accumulated wisdom of my twenty-five years. Wanda
looked at me like she didn't quite understand. Then she pointed to a
set of well-worn road cases, for keyboards and drums. Still I didn't
get it. Was I expected to provide a musical interlude, to "bang the
drum" of good study habits, maybe?

I opened the keyboard case, the interior as musty as a crypt. The
flea-bitten Barkley carcass lay crumpled like a deflated Thanksgiv-

ing Day Parade balloon. A set of size-13 clown shoes and a fat suit, stinking of mothballs, rounded out the "body."

The drum case contained the mutt's head, a papier-mâché globe topped off with a mortarboard hat and rotting graduation tassel. Inside the head was a pair of four-fingered paws, mitts that were caked with filth and foul beyond description. This was Barkley the Smart Dog. And Barkley was me.

Still, as a dominatrix, I couldn't help but be impressed. No sadist I knew could have devised a chamber of horrors so punishing. The clown shoes tripped me; the pelt made me swelter. The fat suit swam out around me, two feet in every direction, depriving me of balance and any sense of physical space. I couldn't have touched two paws together, even if I'd wanted to—there are people who have colons cleaner than those mitts.

But the headpiece—that was the real coup de grace. Seems like the previous Barkley had had a slight drinking problem, and so the interior swirled with the age-old fumes of beer and vomitus. The breathing hole, the snout—which doubled as the seeing hole—was sealed tight with airplane glue.

Needless to say, I was a real hit with the kids. Blind, deaf, fat, stumbling, stoned, dressed like a dog, and laden with coloring books, I was a bully's delight. Wanda, bless her soul, did her best to protect me, but once we'd ventured forth into the audience, we were in way over our heads. These were not Catholic-school children like the ones I'd known, terrified into submission; these were some of the hardest cases from the poorest districts in the state, understaffed and overcrowded. In many of these schools, an appearance from Barkley was roughly akin to a papal visitation—in a country where they hate the pope and want to pelt him with crayons, however.

The little savages went apeshit on me. They yanked on my tail; they knocked on my head; they snatched my coloring books and threw them up into the air. One especially overgrown fourth-grader—I swear he was old enough to shave—ripped my left paw clean off and ran into the crowd holding it high like a hunting trophy. He took one whiff and threw it right back. That's when I learned precisely why they equipped this Barkley with an even number of digits. With no middle finger, you can't show the little darlings what you *really* think.

Still, I took it mostly in stride. I figured it was just the price—and the penance—of my double life. Three days a week, nine months of the year; eventually I made the Barkley character my own. I petitioned the school board to let me get his sad carcass laundered, and while I couldn't convince the dry cleaner to "take care" of the mitts, he did manage to mysteriously lose the shoes. These were replaced, on the Board of Ed's dime, with a pair of candy-apple red Doc Martens. I still wear them to this day.

Some Barkley mornings, when my schedule was tight, I had to wear my mistress gear under my street clothes under my dog outfit. And there was a time when that would have made me supremely uncomfortable, not so much physically as mentally. It seemed too much a collision of my two secret worlds, worlds I'd worked hard to keep separate and safe from each other. But now, freely commingling beneath a fetid fat suit and a moldy graduation hat, it seemed to make perfect sense.

My grandmother went to her grave knowing me not as a layabout, a slacker, or—God forbid—a dominatrix, but as Barkley the Smart Dog, beloved by children and gainfully employed. For that and that alone, it was a job well done.

ANYTHING BUT THE BOYFRIEND

One night, as the evening shift filed into Lady Leona's with our usual joie de vivre—or whatever's the opposite of that—we were greeted by a tragic, familiar sight. Slumped on the couch was our newest mistress, Mistress G., choking on mucus and tears and such despair that she could scarcely speak.

Fortunately, she didn't need to—one look, and we had a diagnosis: a boyfriend who objected to her new vocation, and now it was either the dungeon or him. She told him to go fuck himself, and he said fine, he'd rather. We listened attentively and plied her with cocoa. We'd all done time on that couch.

It seems that G. broke the cardinal rule of mistressing: she let her boyfriend sit in on one of her sessions. If only she had thought to consult with her fellow mistresses first, we would have told her that this was a very bad idea indeed.

Sure, it's great to be in love, the world a verdant field of daffodils, the air warm with the secrets you breathe only to each other. And when you're under the covers together, it's quite tempting to tell that other person everything you ever thought, felt, saw, or purchased in bulk. I'm here to tell you: don't. It may *seem* like a good idea. But, like Olestra and KISS reunion tours, it's an idea that works best at the theory stage. Save full disclosure for your shrink, your priest, and/or your diary. If you're a man, you may share with your mistress. If you're a mistress, leave your man at home, and call periodically to make sure he stays there.

Oh, I've seen it happen enough times with novice doms. There you are, all decked out for Satan's Halloween Parade, looking and feeling like one glamorous badass. You're brimming over with new skills and insights, privy to the seriously wicked secrets of otherwise upstanding adults. You spend your entire workday thinking about sex and money and power—life's greatest intrigues.

It's only natural that you'd want to share your new discoveries with an interested listener, preferably someone with whom you share your sex and money, and so on. And your man will listen to it all, I assure you—but not because he's eager to experience your joy as you do. No, he's mining for clues as to how it all relates to him. And that is totally understandable.

To put it another way: You know how it is sometimes, when you have to call in sick to work, but you're not sick *exactly*—fact is, there's a twelve-hour *CHiPs* marathon on cable and your VCR is busted? I don't know about you, but when it comes time to make that call to the big boss, I need to be alone. I just don't like my loved one to hear me lie, because once he's identified the special timbre of that liar voice, he'll always be on the lookout for it. And he'll be sure he's hearing it sometimes, even when I'm not fibbing. But he'll also hear it on those oh-so-rare occasions when I actually am.

In much the same way, your mistress work demands artifice. But here, when there's that willing suspension of disbelief on the client's part, it's not really lying. It's more like theater. Sexual theater. You have your various routines, monologues, personae, just like in everyday life. And since much of it is based upon what you already know—your real-life sexual experiences—there's going to be some overlap in your sessions.

Now, taken on its own merit, that is necessary and good—it's what lends each session your own unique stamp. And every once in a while you'll get a slave that wants another man to witness the proceedings. That's fine too. Make the slave pay well, and make the witness be anyone—I mean *anyone*—other than someone with whom you are currently enjoying sexual relations.

Beware hubris, resist temptation. Bring your boyfriend and you, lady, are screwed. Because this is what will happen. During the course of the session, you will invariably make some move—could be a gesture, could be a certain tone of voice, a turn of phrase—that he will recognize from your private excursions. From here on in, your sincerity—never mind love—will be forever doubted.

He'll wonder how such private phrases can fall so easily from your tongue to the ears of a stranger; he'll think your every gesture is standard operating procedure. Worse, he'll be waiting for that moment to repeat itself when you're in bed together. He may mention it; he may silently fester. But either way, he'll always wonder if you think of him as just another Philip the Ass Guy. And eventually, you'll hear about it.

On a darker note, think about your role as a dominant. You're expected to call the shots and deal out huge doses of sometimes senseless aggression: roles that are, like it or not, primarily identified as male. What dominatrices do, basically, is fluff up the feminine wiles and pump them full of testosterone.

But if you're not naturally in touch with that masculine side, you've got to borrow from somewhere. Or someone. And if that someone happens to be your significant other, and if he happens to witness this, don't think he'll be overjoyed that you're copping his moves. What you perceive as a loving homage to his studly style, he may perceive as mocking his technique. Bad—very, very bad.

But what if you are a frequent visitor to your own dark side, and your basic relationship struggle is keeping those demons safely locked in the root cellar? What if you invite Mr. Wonderful to watch and you unwittingly let slip a glimpse of your Evil Other that he was better off not knowing about? In other words, a side of you that is just not relevant to your wholesome and loving relationship.

Not too long ago, I let a boyfriend sit in on a session that involved Heavy Corporal—lots of pain, severe punishment—and it hurt my boyfriend more than it hurt the hapless slave. I thought I was being smart, assuring him that my job entailed more agony than sex. I figured he could appreciate guts and gore and a good old-fashioned ass-stomping. His deep, perturbed silence told me that I had been gravely mistaken.

When he finally decided to speak to me again, this is what he said: "I can't believe I sleep with someone who is capable of such fathomless cruelty."

Sure, I tried to explain that to a masochist, it was actually a *nice* thing that I had done—kind of like a massage, only harder. Complete consensuality between two adults, both cognizant of safe words (the magic phrase that makes all play immediately cease) and physical limitations.

But it was to no avail. The image was indelibly seared into his brain; it hovered over every argument, fuss, and dispute, unsaid yet palpable—my true nature, the ugly, evil me. All the sweet words and loving phrases were just an expertly crafted cover for the sick sadist I would eventually reveal myself to be.

—

I soon found myself single again. It was the first time I'd had to contend with the specter of paid domination looming over my love life, so I knew I was in for a real treat. But I hadn't realized just how spoiled I'd been, to have had a mate who knew about my job and thought it was funny—that is, until the very end. Back on the market, I soon discovered that the world was full of two types of men: guys who were horrified by my dungeon career, and guys who were looking for a free session. Oh, and also, guys who had problems that no one could fix.

THE TOUPEE'S THE THING

The only two times I've been branded the evil Other Woman, a guy with a bad hairpiece figured somewhere in the picture. One of my "home-wreckings" happened in the dungeon. But due to the sanctity of mistress/client/nosy girlfriend privilege, I'm afraid I can't tell you about that.

The other time, however, happened in my layperson life. I'd just moved out on my boyfriend of three years and into a brand-new apartment. Due to some quirk in the rental code—and the fact that the place had no heat—the rent was next to nothing, so it was the first time in a long time that I'd lived alone. There I was, freshly single, swinging wildly between the postbreakup poles of despair and exhilaration. As far as I knew, there was only one thing that could soothe my tender, half-broken heart: casual sex.

The very first weekend of my great liberation, I found myself at a party across town. A half dozen cocktails into the evening, I had located my prey. Bryan, or Ryan—it was a really loud party—was a remarkable man in no way whatsoever. The deal was sealed over a couple of shots of Jaegermeister when he asked if he might "walk me home." I knew for a fact that he lived next door; it was a come-on so clear not even a blushing virgin could miss it.

Unfortunately for him, the walk was long and sobering; by the time we'd reached my street, all desire had drained from me like beer from a leaky barrel. Call it perfunctory politeness, but I invited him upstairs anyway. I kept the conversation to topics so dry and lust-busting I may as well have been sitting there picking my nose.

Ever the gracious hostess, I twisted open a bottle of warm Asti Spumante that had been shoring up the kitchen cabinets since before I'd moved in. Not because I was expecting it to rekindle the fires of desire, but because my sense of fair play had been forged by years of faithful game-show viewing. If he wasn't going to make it to the Final Jeopardy of sexual congress, I should at least send him off with a year's supply of Turtle Wax.

Perhaps more significant, it was the first time I'd ever felt real dominatrix attitude spilling over into my personal life. That's right, the mistress in me was beginning to really enjoy the look of chump frustration on the guy's face, a look I'd first detected when I'd led him past all the hot copulation spots—the bedroom, the sofa—and into the harsh, bare-bulbed reality of my frigid spinster's kitchen.

It was the look of a man who'd realized too late that he wasn't getting laid but who, through some biological imperative, was going to attempt that desperate upstream paddle anyway.

I was right in the midst of a monologue concerning the relative merits of safflower oil versus canola (I'm canola, all the way) when he tipped his glass suggestively and made this crude segue.

"Say, Robin, do you know any . . . tricks?"

"You mean like card tricks? Parlor tricks? Huh?"

"I mean tricks like this." And with that, he reached up, unfastened his hair, and flung it at me. It skidded across the table, through a puddle of Spumante and a rancid pat of butter. Then it landed in my lap like the pelt of a dead, greasy animal. I shrieked and kept on shrieking.

"You should see the look on your face," he said, laughing. "It's priceless."

I picked up his toupee and tucked it into his jacket. It peeked out from his pocket like a little brown hanky. "I think it's time we called it a night."

You'd think that would have been the end of it, but then came the parade of answering-machine messages, sure as the morning after. Pleading messages, desperate messages, and finally, messages of bitter accusation. We were like an old married couple by then. Finally he got me on the phone.

"You just don't like me because I don't have hair," he whined.

I tried to explain—tactfully, of course—that I'd dated men in all stages of hair-having, and that it was the fact that he was a toupee-thrower, not a toupee-wearer, that had been his undoing. Of course, being a freak and a loser and a whiny-message-leaver hadn't helped his case much either, and I told him that too.

But I didn't have the heart to mention that he'd been selected, initially, not for genetics but for convenience, and that he'd lost his chance long before he'd flipped his wig, so to speak. I just didn't think we needed to go there.

"So is this a thing, or what?" he demanded. "Are we going to see each other again?"

"Absolutely not."

"So this is goodbye, then?"

"Yes," I replied. "And by the way, I happen to know *many* tricks."

But that wasn't the end of Bryan-Ryan. About four months later, I was at my local health-food store, enjoying a carrot juice and shooting the shit with the juice girl, Kelly, an old friend of mine. Midway through our conversation, this very precisely made-up woman who'd been listening in—and making no pretense about it—sidled up to me.

"Are you *Robin*?" she asked, emphasizing my name as if it were an institution, like Madonna, or Satan.

"I am."

"And do you know a guy named Bryan O'Ryan?"

This I really had to think about. "Well, I did meet a guy at a party once," I said, trying to be helpful. "I think his name was Bryan. Or Ryan. Or something."

"Bryan O'Ryan is my fiancé," she said sharply. "And you'd better just stay away from him." At that, she turned on her heel and marched off.

I was stunned. "Well, tell your *fiancé* to keep his *hair* to himself!" was all I could think of to say.

Walking home, the situation became suddenly clear to me. Whereas my little tête-à-tête with Bryan-Ryan had been a nonevent to me, it had obviously loomed large in his relationship with this smug little missy. God only knows what he must have told her, or why.

Was it a case of prenuptial cold feet that had led him to confess to something that had never even happened? Or maybe she was the repeat cheater, and I was just a name plucked out of nowhere to help him save face. Perhaps, even, this was some little lovers' game they played, a *Who's Afraid of Virginia Woolf?* with a made-up mistress rather than an imaginary child.

Suddenly I could hear my name hurled and unfurled across tabletops and bridal shops, spat out by one or the other in anger, accusation, recrimination, remorse. "I swear to God she meant nothing to me!" cries Bryan-Ryan, banished to the couch.

"Who?" she yells tearfully.

"You know who. *Robin.*"

"I told you I never want to hear that name again!" And she storms out of the bedroom and starts clubbing him ferociously with a throw pillow. She leaves him lying there, alone, knowing in his heart that he was being punished, not for a night of sex that never happened, but for telling a lie that could never be untold.

I can't say I wasn't pleased to have been cast in such a lofty role. The unwitting villainess in someone else's soap opera; I was the home-wrecker, the temptress—and to think, I hadn't even gotten my hands dirty. I was so tickled with my new station in life that I started wearing my mistress clothes outside the dungeon and all around my small town. [http://www.hobokeni.com/slideshow.html] The blood-red talons, the pointy shoes, the high-collared cape—this was how you'd find me attired in the laundromat, at the dog run, and yes, even while enjoying a carrot juice at the health-food store. But that's still not the end of the story. About a month or so after *that,* I came across a photograph of Bryan-Ryan and his betrothed in the "Weddings and Engagements" section of the local newspaper. Maybe it was just because of what I knew about them, but I couldn't help noticing that she seemed to be clinging to him a bit more emphatically than the rest of the wives-to-be, her arms around his neck like a noose. Also, Bryan-Ryan had ditched the rug and was staring back at me, bald as a planet.

I took the absence of toupee as a symbol of the new honesty between them. It seemed as though they had finally worked things out, and I was happy for them, two fucking psychos who deserved each other. And me, looming in the background, an ever-present threat, the evil Other Woman of fiction and fantasy.

HOWIE, CAN YOU HEAR ME?

L ike most people, I keep a mental résumé of things I've done—experiences and accomplishments, assorted dirty deeds—of which I'm perhaps a little too proud. I've seen the Australian Outback and I've hallucinated on absinthe; also, I can roller-skate backward. And like any good résumé, these credentials tend to get, well, exaggerated as the years go by.

At the same time, the list of things I've missed out on—either through fate or fear—is much more extensive, and certainly more telling. For instance, I've come *this* close to meeting Cher, my favorite celebrity, and I'm just beginning to accept the fact that I'll probably never skate in the Roller Derby. And just the other week, there was another depressing addendum to my sheet of also-rans: the Howard Stern *Private Parts* premiere party.

Getting in never seemed like a sure thing. But I had this slave, Marty, an entertainment lawyer, who was owed a favor by a colleague, who happened to have VIP passes and some kind of flu. Now, Marty is a brilliant bullshitter—hence his professional success—but when he rolled up in front of the dungeon in a stretch limo, totally tuxedoed, I started to think he actually might have come through this time. Well, let's just say that I had a little growing up to do!

I won't bore you or aggravate myself by relaying Marty's bullshit litany as we traversed the perimeter of the event, searching for the alleged assistant who held the keys to our VIP sliver of Howard's kingdom. In that mob, we would have had just as much luck finding two men who'd never fantasized about lesbians.

Finally, Marty jumped ship, spitting and grumbling, to storm the gates and see what was going on. I poured myself another drink and settled into the sad fact that not only was it all over, but that the evening he'd promised had probably never existed in the first place.

Through a slit in the tinted window, I watched him disappear into the crowd. To console myself, I picked up his Motorola—he'd conveniently left it sitting on the seat—and called the one person who could remind me that my life had once been rich and exciting and full of adventure: my Outback friend, Glen, who lives in Sydney. I don't talk to him that often, because it's so expensive, so we had a lot of catching up to do.

I didn't make the *Private Parts* party. But that's not to say I've never come close to rubbing elbows with Howard. In fact, I probably got closer on my own than I ever would have with Marty and his VIP lies. Trouble is, I don't remember too much of that night.

It was 1986, a dismal, uninspired year. The *Challenger* exploded, Reagan was still president, and I had another long year at St. Aggie's to look forward to. Wham! was splitting up and that didn't help matters any.

But then, something fun, something meaningful happened—a little-known event attended by a select one hundred people. Like a Woodstock hippie, it is a point of pride to say that I was there, and that the experience changed me—into a sodden, tampon-throwing drunk, but that, too, I consider a badge of honor. To borrow a quote: If you can remember the Howard Stern prom, you probably weren't there.

I was seventeen years old, working at a jewelry store where a bunch of similarly disaffected teens prescribed S-chains, claddagh rings, and Colibri lighters to a working-class and welfare clientele that could ill afford them. But whatever; when you're pulling down $5.25 an hour, you've got little inclination to ponder the Big Picture. My friends worked there. There was a Carvel next door. And we got to tune in to Howard every afternoon.

At the time, Howard wasn't a morning guy, much less a cultural icon; he'd just moved from WNBC to the 2:00–6:00 p.m. slot at K-rock. And while his fan base was growing, his was still a cult status; huge fame among a rabid few who felt that they alone could appreciate him.

Like us, for instance; four high-school kids from Jersey City. So when Howard announced that he was throwing a mock senior prom, we knew there was no way that we—the devoted curators of his myth and brilliance—would stand him up.

Besides, I knew it was the closest I was going to get to a corsage that year. The Stern prom sounded like just the thing: a guaranteed pageant of vulgarity for anyone who was either too cool to attend his own prom, too much of a loser to get a date for it, or someone who affected the attitude of the former because he suspected he might be the latter. The four of us—Fletcher, Steve D., Charise, and me—represented the full range of that spectrum.

We were going in style, no question about it. First we needed a ride. Turned out that Black Rod, this ex-biker and our UPS guy, moonlighted at a limo company. He agreed to take us for cheap as long as we took care of his head and he didn't have to clean out the car beforehand. He'd been hired to chauffeur for a real prom, and wasn't about to clean up puke and used prophylactics in the one-hour gap between their big night and ours.

Steve D. and Fletcher rented tuxedos: powder blue, with ruffles and cummerbund, a style statement only slightly more refined than the tuxedo T-shirt. I'd like to say that our fashion choices were made in the spirit of irony, but I really can't be sure. Charise had her shoes dyed to match her purse, which matched her eyeshadow, lipliner, and blush; all were a painful shade of crimson that most people associate with clown noses, or panic buttons. Intended as a joke, it would have been hysterical, except that Charise was a bona fide Jersey Girl and took her color coordination very seriously.

Then she turned her sights on me, the sartorially challenged. One sweltering afternoon, we picked up a Cookie Puss from next door and hurried it back to her house. Generous soul that she was, she flung open her closet to me, but nothing quite worked. [http://www.inthe80s.com] Granted, the eighties were hard on all of us, but they seemed to have been especially unkind to Charise. Material Girl lace and Thompson Twins brocade, Bananarama spandex, with a special emphasis on the belly cutout and the jaunty straw hat.

Finally I let her pick out a dress. Except it wasn't really a dress; it a swath of fabric upholstering the two colossal shoulder pads that jutted from my neck like twin wedges of Camembert.

We stared at me, and my new build, in the mirror. "*Totally* excellent," she said. "Let's accessorize."

"With what? A football?"

Eventually, I found my dress, but not through Charise, and not without consequences. I got it from this girl at school, Dani, in exchange for the answers on a social-studies final. It was black, strapless, unadorned, and tight as a rubber band. Perfect. However, it also carried a dishonorable legacy, which Dani warned me about.

"Every time I wear it, I wake up with the wrong guy," she confided.

"You mean a guy who's not your boyfriend?"

"No, I mean like a teacher."

Like so many nights that end in regret, it seemed to start out innocently enough. Our boss, Jimmy "the Jeweler" Mancini, an avid Howard fan, threw us a little send-off party at the store. Jimmy was one of those *fun* grown-ups; sort of like our kindly but corrupting uncle, and he put out quite a spread: cold cuts, vino, Thai stick, condoms. He was also an amateur photographer, took lots of pictures.

You know, all the requisite send-off stuff, cheek-kissing and corsage-pinning in every possible combination.

At the time, nothing seemed amiss. It wasn't until Jimmy developed the photos that we noticed my corsage had been weighing down the front of my dress. And there it was—my right tit, clearly exposed, the nipple winking daintily atop a pink carnation cloud. Also, Fletcher's fly was gaping open, something that had escaped our notice as well.

Then there was the five-dollar bill we found in the back of the limo. Flecked with dried blood, it should have been a bit of a tipoff. But nooo, we were young; we were immortal. We thought it was *cool*.

Steve D. started rolling up the bill so we could enjoy some of the "cocaine" he'd been saving especially for the occasion. It was the kind of very cut crap they sell only to high-school students, the perfect complement to those dyed-spaghetti bits we knew as "mescaline."

When they couldn't find a surface on which to lay out "lines," Charise donated her powder compact. The mirror was cracked, but that didn't stop us from passing it through the privacy partition to Black Rod. A bloody bill and a cracked mirror? Even when conjured on the New Jersey Turnpike, Rod knew bad juju when he saw it. He passed it right back to us, untouched, sealed tight the partition, and wouldn't speak to us for the rest of the evening.

Me, I stuck with the vodka—about three tumblers of it. I was new to drinking, apparently as new as Fletcher was to mixology. Thanks to the coke, however, what he lacked in experience he more than made up for in enthusiasm. So as long as he kept mixing, I kept tossing them back.

By the time we hit the South Amboy exit, I'd downed close to a fifth of Wolfschmidt, Fletcher had a torrential nosebleed, and Charise had nearly put an eye out with her mascara wand. Steve D., meanwhile, was on the floor with the fiver, vacuuming the carpet for any stray grains of blow. "Lift your feet, lift your feet," he exhorted us, like a coke-addled grandma, each time he passed by.

We rolled into the Club Bene parking lot and tumbled out of our limo. We made quite an entrance, but it was not elegant; it was Emergency Room. We staggered into the club like accident victims, bleeding and bolstering one another. So I'm afraid I don't have much in the way of first impressions. What I do remember of those first heady moments is that the room was studded not with stars, but with inebriated white trash. Also, forget "Dreams" or "Friendship"; the theme of this prom was clearly "Feminine Hygiene."

Fletcher noticed it first. Desperate for something to stanch his nosebleed, he reached up and grabbed one of the streamers that ribboned the room from end to end. It ripped easily—too easily, like toilet paper. In fact, it *was* toilet paper. Somehow this set off a piñatalike reaction of party favors dropping from the rafters—jockstraps, panty liners, tampons, enema hoses, and Fiesta condoms, one of which landed in Charise's big hairdo and stuck there, like a fly in a spider's sticky web.

Eventually we found a booth and poured ourselves into it. The table's centerpiece was a bouquet of tampons that flowered open, nodding like tulips on their cardboard stems. I leaned against the wall. The paneling was oddly soft and cushiony, as though Howard had anticipated my need for a headrest. I pulled back and looked at my pillow: a Stayfree Overnight maxi.

Then, just as night follows day, it was toilet-bowl time. I don't know how I found the powder room, I'm just grateful that I found it on time. Here I remember three distinct events: puking into the toilet; Charise holding back my bangs as I puked into the toilet; Charise leaving, and me puking through a scrim of hair.

When that got tedious, I found myself a nice, relatively unused stretch of counter space, climbed up, and settled in for a little nap. I remember waves of women marching into the bathroom, trying to interrupt my rest. The fussy bitches kept asking me to move so they could "freshen their lipstick" and "use the sink." Apparently, I was "in their way." *If I wanted to pass out in a powder room full of cunts,* I grumbled to myself, *I could have gone to my own prom.*

Some time later, Charise came and retrieved me. Something was about to happen, she told me, something I wouldn't want to miss. It was time for Howard Stern and Robin Quivers to select the King and Queen of the Prom. There were several contenders for the throne; the winners would be the couple willing to perform the most outrageous stunt for the rest of us.

While I'd been sleeping, Fletcher had been busily perfecting his act. Using the disposable applicator, he deftly slid a Tampax, Slender Regular, up his afflicted nostril. But before we could convince him to get up on stage, he was quickly outdone by the rest of the talent. As the entire prom looked on, a woman from Canarsie took her six-inch stiletto heel and stuck it up her date's ass. This was years before my time in the dungeon; I'd never seen anything like that before. The crowd went wild. We threw tampons and maxis and jockstraps at the King and Queen as they were crowned, robed, and sceptered.

Then the prom was over. Steve D. and Fletcher gallantly carried me back to the limo, tucking me under their arms like a rolled-up carpet, or a battering ram. They'd had a pretty rough night too. Steve D. had lost his cummerbund and Fletcher had bled all over his ruffled shirt—both rented, both ruined.

But we weren't the only casualties. All around us, people were limping along in groups of two and three, like those battle-weary patriots in *The Spirit of '76.* You could practically hear the tootling of the fife as they helped one another back to their limos, holding their heads, clutching their spoils. We'd made it to the prom, and we'd made it *through* the prom. All that was left were the stories we'd tell.

The next afternoon, we regrouped at Jimmy's Jewels—not to work, but to let him taunt and treat our hangovers, and to tune in to Howard's postprom show. The hope was that we'd get some insider details, maybe even hear about things we'd been too incapacitated to notice. But what we got was better than that. Steve D. was referred to as "that moron looking for coke"; Fletcher as "that guy with the tampon up his nose." Charise, I believe, was dubbed "some big-haired Stop sign."

"And what about the girl that was passed out in the ladies' room all night," Howard said.

Then Robin chimed in: "Yeah, what was her problem, anyway?"

"I think she was drunk. People kept trying to wake her up, but she wouldn't leave."

Howard had seen us! He had insulted us! It was hard not to notice—and I didn't want to gloat—that although I'd clocked the least waking prom time, in the end it was I who scored the most Howard airtime. Not just some offhand sobriquet, but a genuine call-and-response. A dialogue! This was better than anything I could have hoped for.

I never saw much of Steve D. and Fletcher and Charise after that. I'd like to say it had something to do with prom night, like hostages or prisoners of war who don't keep in touch because they can't deal with reliving the intensity of the experience.

But it was nothing like that. We were kids and it was summer; for some of us, college was right around the corner. The only thing I regret is that I have no way to confirm that the night actually happened, no one to reminisce with. Thanks to my topless "overexposure," Jimmy had respectfully destroyed the photographs, so there's no evidence, either. Was it just another "Wedding in Brownsville," a ballroom full of ghosts? Does anybody out there remember the Howard Stern prom?

PART III

THE COOLDOWN

LEAVING THE PLANTATION

I'd made it maybe halfway through my second year of mistressing when things started going seriously downhill. It was the classic sophomore slump: I was losing interest in my studies, and yet saw no end in sight. Also, there were certain extenuating circumstances.

Lady Leona, our not-so-esteemed boss, had been out of town—and out of our hair—for months and months. She'd fallen in love with a guy twelve years her junior, the heir to a sugarcane fortune, a white-suited South African lad who bore a startling resemblance to Simon Le Bon, the lead singer of Duran Duran. We called him Plantation Boy.

The sole focus of P-Boy's life seemed to be letting Leona support him while they waited for his crops to come in. Meanwhile, on Leona's dime, they hopped from cruise ship to cruise ship, taking care of important plantation business in places such as Puerto Rico, Barbados, and—this I found telling—the Cayman Islands.

I don't know much about growing seasons or sugarcane futures, but I sure know the sickly sweet aroma of a scam when I smell it. Soon enough—and too soon for everyone's taste—Leona was back in our midst. She was far too proud to tell us what had really happened, and somehow this steel-willed dignity made her unusually sympathetic.

So we listened politely and cheered her on as she spun tale after tale of living high on Plantation Boy's fortune, clucking our tongues in grim understanding when she told us that even though he spoiled her rotten and treated her like a queen, in the final analysis, she was too much woman for him to handle. Apparently, she'd needed a Plantation Man.

But our sisterhood was short-lived. Powered by the twin turbines of heartache and humiliation—and probably deeply in debt—Leona threw herself into running the dungeon. To help expand the business, Leona hired a consultant—not a managerial whiz or an asset analyst, but a Santeria priestess with psychic abilities.

This woman made two prophecies: First, there was drug use on the premises; second, girls were stealing clients away from the dungeon and seeing them privately, to avoid paying the house half to Leona.

Of course you didn't need a psychic friend to make that prediction about almost any dungeon anywhere. But Leona's "seer" did provide details so stunningly accurate that we began to suspect the phone in the mistress lounge was tapped.

To recoup her divined loss, Leona started to enforce a strict schedule of fines (lateness, $20; out of uniform, $30; forgetting to bring condoms, $25) and treated us all to a 10 percent pay cut. She claimed that this was the only way she could afford to keep the Reformatory open. Naturally, this only caused the stealing to intensify—proof that no matter what your milieu, people will always live down to the expectations set for them.

Up until this point, Leona's attitude toward me had been strictly hands-off; I made her plenty of money with a minimum of drama, and she was pragmatic enough not to fuck with the formula. But then she took me aside and told me that because I earned outside income from my column—and since many of my columns were inspired by her establishment, though she'd never actually read them—she felt that I should contribute a greater percentage than the other girls.

Now, asking us to dig into our pockets was one thing; helping the business, from which we'd already stolen so much, seemed within the realm of reason. And it was easy enough to circumvent the sanctions, so no one really cared. But the sheer suggestion that I dig into my own life on her behalf—that was something I wouldn't even dignify with a refusal. I held my tongue; I calmly accepted the signs— it was time to start getting out.

But I didn't just pack my bags—that would have been hasty and unwise. Nor did I openly challenge Leona—that would only have made her more determined to shake me down. Instead, I just let her forget about it, something I knew would happen as soon as some easier mark presented itself.

I didn't intend to give up mistressing; I just didn't want to let so much of my income be dependent upon Leona's dungeon—and whims. So I decided to see my departure not as an incident, but as a process. A process by which I gradually lured some of my wealthiest, most trustworthy clients out of Leona's place and into the fifth-floor walkup I shared with my best friend, Desi. Meanwhile, I'd maintain a modest presence at Leona's—it was a great place to cultivate new clients.

For weeks, Desi and I had been talking about setting up shop, and she was more than agreeable. For one thing, she was rarely home— her boyfriend owned a luxury loft in SoHo. Also, it was an easy way for her to make some no-obligation mistressing money; every so often, I'd hire her to sit in on a session when one of my clients asked for an inexperienced participant. Fortunately for both of us, my most loyal follower happened to be that connoisseur of innocence, that gourmand of green, Chester the Molester.

CHESTER SAVES THE DAY—SORT OF

I've never exchanged sex for money—not in the traditional sense, anyway—and it's not because I've never had the opportunity. Nor do I have any problem with the idea; in the course of the day, we all hand over pieces of ourselves far more precious than a few minutes' worth of friction, things you can hardly price. There are worse things you can sell someone than an orgasm.

No, there's a more practical reason I've never done the deed. See, I understand that when you fuck for bucks, it's not really the john that you're having sex with. You're actually making love to the security, comfort, and ease that the money will bring you. You're making love to that which will save you from desperation and ruin and the thwarting of your dreams. In my case, the stakes have simply never been that high, and so I've never met a lover I couldn't resist.

But that's not to say I've never been tempted. In particular, there was that tricky transition in the beginning of the year, when I was halfway between working at Leona's and striking out on my own. One of the clients I'd stolen from Leona's was Chester the Molester— the wealthy cradle robber who liked to corrupt the post-teenybopper set. At twenty-five, I was about as "post" as it gets, but it was a lucrative gig and he bought my act, so I figured that as long as he didn't cut me in half and count my rings, everything would be okay.

It was a bitter, bitter February, freeze-ass cold. Desi and I were living on the Lower East Side, in one of those buildings that had gotten lost in the co-op/condo conversion frenzy, and so was left a half-gentrified tenement. We were not so much living there as squatting, except that we were dumb enough to actually pay rent, and way too much of it.

The wind whistled, the pipes froze; every other morning, we would find a thin sheet of piss-tinted ice in the toilet bowl. Some nights we had to huddle together like sheep beneath sheets and blankets and throw rugs, but that wasn't the worst of it. See, we had this radiator that clanged and banged but never threw heat, except during those odd occasions when I happened to have some unfortunate client secured to it. *Then* it burned hot as Satan's pitchfork.

It quickly became apparent that the more clients we could lure to our place, the better our chances of surviving that hard winter. *Lure* was the operative word—we had to make it seem as though there were added benefits to choosing our hovel, with its authentic privations, over the comfort and fabricated tortures of Leona's place. We had to figure out what the client really wanted, and imply that somehow, our place was where that fantasy would finally be realized. In the case of Chester, his most heartfelt desire was to watch me get it on with one of my "teenybopper" girlfriends.

Desi was my age but, due to good genetics and a two-hour-a-day workout, looked about sixteen. She was also an up-and-coming film director; we were in the midst of negotiating a low-six-figure deal, but could barely afford the shoe leather to hoof it up to our attorney's office. So Desi was the only woman I could think of who was as desperate, hungry, and determined as I was. She was also the only other woman cold enough to roll around with me in the throes of fabricated lust.

So one afternoon, I yanked off one of my Thinsulate gloves and dialed Chester's pager. Once he saw the number, and the special code that indicated that Desi was on the premises, he called me back quick. "Is your little friend ripe for picking?" he panted into the phone.

"I think that might be the case," I replied, trying to sound furtive. "And is your little playmate getting hot?"

I glanced over at Desi, who was desperately doing ab crunches, her Adidas planted between the rungs of the cold, dead radiator. "Things might warm up if maybe you came over," I confided through chattering teeth.

Thus Chester quickly laid out his plan for me. Just as he was making the approach in his BMW, he would dial our number from his car phone, letting it ring once. That was my cue to send Desi out of the house on some errand, and I would let him in the door and into our closet. There he would squat, jerking off into our pantyhose, as I expressed my long-hidden feelings of lust to Desi. At the precise moment that our passion erupted into a frenzied bout of mutual cunnilingus, Chester, Child Molester, would make his presence known. I hung up the phone and relayed this information to Desi.

"D'ya really think Chester expects us to eat pussy?" Desi asked dubiously.

"Guess he knows we gotta eat *something,*" I replied.

Then Desi and I hatched our own plan, which had to do with our upstairs neighbors, Rodrigo and Marta, the Portuguese hatebirds.

Desi and I were intimately familiar with the tide of their ill-fated romance due to a sixteen-by-sixteen-inch chasm in our ceiling, their floor. We could see right up into their bathroom, just as they could look down into ours, and every once in a while some of their possessions—a hairbrush, a carving knife, a crack stem—would fall through.

It was not so much that we minded eavesdropping on their horrible bouts (though the sight of Marta banging Rodrigo's head into their toilet tank did leave me constipated for days). No, it was the fact that their endless carryings-on competed unfavorably with the beatings being handed out in our flat; it made my paying, willing victims uneasy. Something needed to be done—and I'm not talking about calling the cops, who stopped coming. What Desi and I wanted was to get that damn ceiling fixed.

Enter Chester the Molester, all duded up like he's the one who's gonna get laid. As Desi practiced wind sprints up and down the stairwell, I stashed him in the closet, where he nestled precariously atop a stack of videotapes. Just as I was closing the closet door, out peeped his eager, bald head. "If you need any help finding her little clitty," he offered, "I'm here for you."

I threw a ripped pair of panties at him. "Good to know, Chester."

When Desi returned, I led her into the living room and took her cold hand in mine. "Desiree, lately I have detected a feeling between us that is more than friendship," I began, "and even though we're just two teenage girls, I think we owe it to ourselves to, you know, get it on."

"Oh, Ruby," she exclaimed, "even though we're both virgins, I think I know desire when I feel it. Kiss me! Kiss me as only a young and nubile nymphet can kiss another! Right here! Right now!"

And then, just as we were about to make contact, so help me, Chester came half-stumbling, half-charging out of the closet as if propelled by the urgency of his own erection. He stood before us, pumping it in his fist, panties over his face. We pretended to look surprised. It was a once-in-a-lifetime shot, and I know Desi wished we had a camera handy.

From there, things devolved into a more basic S&M scenario. We trussed Chester to the radiator—leaving his jack-off hand free, naturally—and huddled on the couch, shivering and pretending to flirt with each other, our breath crystallizing in the air. When it became obvious that the heat wasn't going to come on, Desi declared that she'd feel much more amorous if only she could get warm.

"I could eat your pussy," Chester suggested brightly. "That would make you warm as toast."

No, Desi said, it wasn't the cold exactly. It was the fearsome draft. We led him to it. "See," I said. "The people upstairs can watch us pee and stuff."

"It's almost perverted," Desi chimed in.

Chester yanked away thoughtfully. "Think they'd be interested in selling that unit?" he asked.

So we made Chester call Tomassi, our one-eyed junkie janitor. It was fascinating to witness Chester's captain-of-industry persona overtake the fat, naked, pud-pulling pervert that we knew: "Yeah, we got a drywall situation in 18E needs to get some action. . . . Needta review the service contract pronto."

"Service contract, my left nut!" Tomassi replied. "Are you fucking crazy?! This is a fucking shit-hole tenement, asshole." And so on.

So our apartment never got warm (unless you count July, when it baked), our ceiling never got fixed, Rodrigo went to jail, and Marta, the real batterer, went free. Chester never gave us the money he promised, our lawyer never got paid, and our project fell through. Tomassi went on methadone, and Desi and I never had sex—together, that is. But spring eventually came and new endeavors bloomed and blossomed, and neither thanks nor blame is due Chester, Child Molester.

———

Both of my fantasy-oriented careers—mistressing and writing—were progressing nicely. I'd managed to whittle down my hours at Leona's to one or two shifts a week, and I'd just been voted "Best *New York Press* Columnist" in the paper's annual readers' poll. But then real life—in the form of a miserable health crisis—stepped in, and I was knocked out of commission for the next five weeks.

RX FOR PAIN

Normally, I have a pretty low opinion of women who write about their vaginas. It seems like a topic best reserved for lovers, doctors, close friends, women's magazines, and good, graphic pornography. Anywhere else, I positively cringe for my sisters. It's a lot like watching your kid cousin get drunk for the first time and strip at the family reunion: She wants to demonstrate that she's not a little girl anymore; everyone else wants to cover her with a coat. Normally, it's a subject I'd never touch in these pages. But there haven't always been normal times at the Ruby household, and so I offer you this cautionary tale.

One late-winter afternoon I was sitting at my desk, writing this column. I stood up and noticed that my legs were covered in blood, as if I'd taken a bullet in the thigh. I made my way to the bathroom, where I collapsed on the floor. Eventually, the agony subsided. I cleaned up in the shower, got dressed to go out, and skipped off into the night.

These attacks were nothing new to me. I'd been living with them for the last week or so, when they'd strike every afternoon, sure as soap operas. I'd gotten so accustomed that I'd started scheduling my day around them, not making appointments with clients or editors or friends between the hours of 4:00 and 6:00 p.m., when my chin had a date with my knees.

Actually going to the doctor was something that simply hadn't occurred to me. I am young, and therefore immortal, and more important, uninsured. In my quest for quality birth control, I'd just sunk close to a thousand bucks into my reproductive system, and I'd be damned if I was going to see my investment go down the toilet, so to speak.

The next day, dinner with the family. I was holding it together pretty well through the turkey and the fixings, but the pain was in the mail, that much was for sure. By the time dessert rolled around it felt like I was getting raped by a birdcage. I excused myself and staggered out of sight, assuming the position on the carpet at the top of the stairs.

Some time later, I opened my eyes to see my family looming over me in a semicircle, a strange little Sunday tableau. My mom, who thinks every physical ailment is gas, suggested Kaopectate. My dad, who thinks every physical ailment is cancer, shuffled his feet nervously, hoping against hope that I would use the word *period* or *cramps,* so that he might slink decorously away.

My brother, who had no idea of what he'd just walked in on, stood clutching the turkey wishbone. The snapping of the bone is perhaps the last vestige of sibling rivalry between us, and it's as bitterly contested today as it was when we were kids (mainly because he's a big cheater). Apparently we weren't going to let a few lousy death throes get in the way of a time-honored tradition.

For a moment, that cursed bone looked for all the world like my Ortho ParaGard Copper-T 380 IUD, the source of my agony. He held it out to me, already enjoying his victory, and I gave it a vengeful snap. A vicious spasm shot through my entire reproductive tract. Defeated again.

Looking back, it's hard to imagine how I could think that having a two-inch shard of copper embedded in my uterus would be a hassle-free form of pregnancy prevention. But I had my reasons, and at the time, they seemed sound. I'd learned early on that the world of birth control is fraught with greed and misinformation, dubious devices and slipshod services. Back in high school, my girlfriends and I were regular patients at a place called Options, the women's free clinic around the block from St. Aggie's. Believe me, everything they say about promiscuous Catholic-school girls is true; by 3:00 p.m., the waiting room was a veritable sea of plaid skirts—and we represented only the responsible ones. Around school, the clinic was known as "eighth period," or, in more desperate cases, "no period."

It was there that I received a crash course in my reproductive rights. I have the right to go on the Pill; to get fat, to get acne, to get depressed, to get headaches, to get potentially fatal blood clots to the brain and a three-inch-long chin hair that sprouts in the middle of the night. Ditto Norplant, ditto Depo-Provera.

I have the right to talk a guy into using a condom. I have the right to foams, jellies, creams, and spermicides, which have been proven to kill one's appetite for oral sex far more reliably than they will kill actual sperm. I have the right to a diaphragm and to the urinary tract infection that it will invariably inspire, and a right to all subsequent yeast infections induced by bladder-infection antibiotics.

That said, wanna fuck?

Now, I'm no conspiracy nut, but I'm starting to suspect that this whole mess was originally invented by some bitter old asshole who couldn't get laid and wanted to see to it that the rest of us never got any either. Or worse, that the whole point is to just give up and start populating the world willy-nilly.

But what really bothers me is that what are considered "acceptable" side effects in the world of birth control—where the onus is on the woman—would never be tolerated in a medication intended for the general population.

If I didn't know any better, I'd start to get the message that sex equals suffering and that sidestepping motherhood requires some kind of punishment. That wanting to have sex for sex's sake is a brazen act, more than a girl should ask for. If I refuse to nurse a child, I will be forced to nurse myself.

Of course, that's a message I refused to accept. The lousy treatment I was accustomed to wasn't specific to federally funded inner-city clinics; it was the same game in private practice, except that I was paying for it.

Eventually, counterintuition kicked in. I'd come to the conclusion that if your doctor doesn't want you to have it, it's probably a good thing. And that's when I decided that I had to have an IUD. Who knows? Maybe it's the best-kept secret in the birth-control biz. And I wouldn't be talked out of it.

When they told me that bedouins would stuff pebbles into the uteruses of their camels, to keep them from getting pregnant on long journeys, I thought, *How quaint.* When they told me that no one really knows how the IUD works, I thought, *Well, maybe there's something to be said for a little bit of mystery.*

When they told me I might suffer anemia, backache, fainting, spotting, cramps—to name but a few—I figured it was no worse than what I'd already suffered through other methods. When they told me that the IUD could lead to ectopic pregnancy, infertility, or death, I thought, *Propaganda! Scare tactics!* When my doctor told me that overall, he just couldn't recommend it, I said, basically, that we should forget about me as a sexually active single woman, and start thinking of me as what I really was—a paying customer. *Here's my eight hundred bucks. Bring it on.* [http://www.gynpages.com/ultimate]

The first week I spent doubled over on the couch. I figured my body was just getting used to it, an adjustment period that was to be expected. The second week, I took it out for a road test, and another four days on the couch ensued. I figured that that was just getting used to having sex, IUD-style. The third week was the week of my daily 4:00 to 6:00 p.m. pain siesta. In terms of lost time, lost wages, pain and suffering, and miserable quality of life, it beat out, by an overwhelming margin, all other methods of birth control combined. And the fuck of it all is that I still didn't want to give it up.

Looking back, I think I hung on the same way that some people stay with a lousy job or a bad habit or a boyfriend who treats you badly. I made excuses for it, I prayed it would change, I thought maybe the problem would just go away by itself. Not because I thought I deserved it, but because I didn't want to face the fact that there might not be anything better out there.

And in the wee hours that followed that fateful family dinner, when I was writhing in pain and spiking a fever, piled into the backseat of my dad's car, heading to the hospital, I was still hoping we could manage to work it out.

The funny thing was, the moment the hospital came into view, most of my visible symptoms—the shivering, the shaking, the pathetic fetal posture—completely vanished. Even the fever was down. Good news for me, sure, but in a place where you basically need to have a bloody ax blade wedged in your forehead to get any attention, a little internal hemorrhaging just wasn't gonna cut it.

My mother, ever the shrewd one, knew this too. "Better start looking bad," she whispered tersely, "or we'll be here until Easter." I obliged with a reenactment of some of the month's worst moments. I collapsed into a seat (the floor was disgracefully filthy); I doubled over onto my side; I moaned and spasmed and clutched at my stomach.

Mom, who is a first-class crusader, screwed on her game face and pounded the receptionist's desk with her fist, like a judge banging a gavel. "That woman is my daughter and she is gravely ill," she said, pointing a finger in my direction. The startled woman looked up from her typewriter. I moaned louder, for effect.

"She is also a columnist for a major newspaper and I suggest that you find her a doctor *immediately!*" I giggled into my sleeve. She's a real panic, my mom.

Whether they feared the wrath of my mighty pen, or whether it just happened to be a slow day for emergencies, I'll never know for certain. As a writer, status is circumstantial. Whereas it may have gotten me some action in Admissions, the payment lady was less than impressed. As soon as she saw what I'd listed as my occupation, she sighed wearily and slid a sheaf of Medicaid forms through the bulletproof glass. She had my deadbeat little number, that was for sure—I may as well have written "pauper," "loser," or "lots of luck collecting."

We settled in and watched the sad parade of urban decay that's probably just business as usual at an inner-city emergency room. Babies cried. Junkies fought over the bathroom. The man sitting downwind of us consumed three cherry Chapsticks in the space of twenty minutes.

But the saddest lot were the emergency room regulars—senior citizens, all lost and forgotten, clutching their possessions in tattered D'Agostino bags—coming in for their weekly pressure check, waiting in line for someone, anyone, to give an ear to their litany of complaints.

Eerier still, they all shared a certain look of frumpy distractedness, a look of yellowing dust-jacket photographs—a look that could only be described as "writerly." Were these men the Mailers, the Fromms, the Vonneguts—minus the book deals?

Finally, my wheelchair arrived, and I was whisked away. Somehow I imagined they might take me someplace special, maybe a ward reserved for victims of sexual mishaps. I'd lie gurney-to-gurney with a guy who had his dick stuck in a vacuum-cleaner hose, a woman who'd autoerotically asphyxiated, a man with a hamster lodged in his colon. Thinking of my predicament as the consequence of bizarre sex play was strangely comforting; thinking of it as the consequence of a barbaric form of birth control was not. Realistically, the only way my IUD had helped thwart conception was by making me too sick for sex—or for anything else, for that matter.

But it wasn't until the nurse checked my vitals that we realized how very far things had gone. My pulse was slow and faint. My pressure was 80 over 50—and definitely not rising. I'd lost so much blood over the last week that I was severely dehydrated and twelve pounds lighter. The blue fingernails suggested anemia; the 100-plus fever, infection. Now it appeared that the only way my IUD had succeeded at keeping me childless was by possibly rendering me sterile, or, if we had waited a couple weeks longer, dead.

So I stepped into a gown and spiked an IV and mounted the stirrups and waited for the gyno to show. He was a nice-enough man, as far as doctors go, firmly focused on the bottom line. Didn't care why or how I'd gotten into this mess; the point was, the IUD was killing me, both literally and figuratively, and it had to come out. He was going to snap on a glove, yank the offending shard, prescribe some antibiotics, and send me on my way.

But then something strange happened, when he was poking around. My mom, who was sitting in the corner, correcting papers, sensed it even before I did. "What's the problem?" she asked.

He frowned and removed his finger. "I don't feel it anywhere."

"So . . . what does that mean?" I asked.

"That means it's probably lost in your system," he replied.

"And what does *that* mean?" asked my mom, who by now was looming over both of us, red pen poised. I only hoped she didn't "correct" the guy before he had a chance to heal me.

"I fear it may have punctured your uterus," he said, jotting something onto my chart. "I fear it may have pierced your rectum."

Now that's trendy, I thought. *A rectum piercing.*

The good doctor spelled out my options. First thing tomorrow, I could go to the office of a colleague of his—he had the proper equipment—and take care of it there. Or I could wait a couple hours and he would operate right here, in the hospital.

He was only telling me this because he knew I had no insurance, being a writer and all that. "Operations are expensive," he said. "And I've got a funny feeling you're not exactly Jackie Collins." He chuckled—a bit too heartily.

Maybe not, I thought. But it doesn't take a Hollywood wife to understand that full anesthesia beats a local and a huge bill from a faceless institution is a bill I won't be losing any sleep over.

I looked him square in the eye. "Money is no object," I said. "Let's operate."

By this time, it was about eleven in the morning. We'd been at the hospital since 5:00 a.m. The OR wouldn't be free till late in the evening. My mom put on her coat to go apprise my dad of the situation; he was sitting outside in the car, patiently working his way through a backlog of *New York Times* crosswords (*28 down: Fretful, in a way*).

I suggested that they just drive off and get themselves some lunch, maybe catch a show, make a fun day of it. No point sitting here with me when all I was good for was sleep. "Are you sure you don't want me to stay here and watch you?" she asked, patting my blue little hand.

"Sure I'm sure," I said cheerily. "Besides, you'll have plenty of time to look at my picture after I'm dead."

The day got worse, and weirder. They'd stripped me of all my earthly possessions—from boots to clothes to contact lenses—and I was now blind as Milton, draped in a gown and tethered to the gyno table by means of an IV drip on a rolling stand.

In the corner of the room, there was a cabinet chock-full of medical supplies, and you know I've always had a huge weakness for anything latex, talcumed, designed to draw blood, or individually wrapped. So I was dying to roll over there and have myself a look, maybe snag some parting gifts from Caligari's cabinet.

Just as I was making the initial attempt, a young nurse came into the room to adjust my IV. She checked my chart. "So you're a writer," she said conversationally. "Is that a hobby or are you someone I might know?"

Now, I've always bristled at that "hobby" business—as if I'd do this for fun and not out of some sick necessity—and I'd had quite enough of being condescended to. So you can blame it on hubris if you like, but Lord help me, I gave up the goods.

"Oh my God! You're Mistress Ruby, and I am your biggest fan!" she exclaimed. "Do you think if I bring you a copy of the paper, you'll sign it for me?" Certainly, I told her, I'd be happy to oblige, if she might also bring a bag and help me lift some stuff from the supply closet. "Oh, you're so funny!" she gushed.

Needless to say, it was the world's worst time to have outed myself. And it was an even worse time, an hour or so later, when I had finally freed myself and was elbow-deep in a drawer full of latex tie-off strips, when the door swung open and the nurse strode in with another of my "biggest fans"—a male nurse this time—in tow. And there I stood, caught in the act, ass out and tangled up in my own IV tubing, like an exhibitionist derelict thief.

He was gracious enough to overlook the small pile of take-home I'd amassed as he enthusiastically shook my free, nonthieving hand; still, it wasn't exactly the way I wanted to meet my public. "I *told* you she was funny," the first nurse said to the second, as if it were an accusation.

Finally it was time to take that long, slow trip to the operating room. As we made the descent into the chilly bowels of the hospital, I could hear the portentous voice-over in my head: *It started out as a routine procedure . . .*

Somehow, word that they had a very low-level celebrity on their hands had spread to the OR team. Fortunately, in the six hours that had elapsed since my "unveiling," they'd lost the thread and didn't know exactly who. Considering that they were getting ready to knock me out, spread my legs, stick a camera and a knife up through my vagina and into my uterus, I opted—since I couldn't salvage my dignity—to at least maintain my anonymity.

"So we hear you're a columnist for a New York newspaper," said the anesthesiologist, as he ran a line into my vein. "Anyone we might know?"

Had this been any other type of situation, I would have thought it great fun to tell them that I was Peyser, or Bushnell, or Isadora the Advice Hippie. But these good doctors had my life in their hands; there was no call for cattiness.

"Goodness, no," I said, as I started slipping away, "it's strictly a hobby."

I figured that was the kind of thing Jackie Collins would have said.

—

Once the doctors desharded me, my recovery was swift and uncomplicated. I took to my couch and observed a strict regimen of *Real World* marathons and *Cosmo* quizzes ("Otter, Snake, or Bear—Find Your Secret Sexual Animal!"). Soon enough, I was back in action. I wouldn't say that I was milking the situation, but I did notice that the sympathy of friends was a healing tonic. The more people marveled at my ordeal, the better I began to feel.

Eventually I broke down and wrote about my IUD debacle for *New York Press*. The response was truly touching. I'd been away from my column for over a month, and my readers had actually been worried about me. The letters, cards, and e-mails poured in—expressing empathy, offering advice, or promising me justice, sometimes even vengeance.

One reader sent me a teddy bear customized with a tiny leather bondage harness; another lawyer client offered to sue my gyno, the hospital, the entire state of New York if necessary. I politely declined, but these gestures more than made up for the indignities of my hospital "outing." *This* was the love of the people, and it felt better than any applause, or recognition, or fame.

JESUS, GRANDMA, AND JOSEPH

L ike some sick, S&M version of a *Seinfeld* character—the Low Talker, the Soup Nazi—Joseph was a closeted Close-Getter. I told you about him some time ago: the Kent-smoking seventies throwback who spent months and months putzing through pointless and boring sessions until the day I cracked and he spilled.

What he *really* wanted, he'd finally confided, was for me to don a nun's habit and catch him masturbating—in the cloakroom, in the corner, at his desk, and so on, amen. Stuff I knew about—more or less—from my own internment in Catholic school.

You understand that it was not the request itself, but his reluctance to reveal it, that threw me. I mean, seriously, what the hell did he think I was doing in that dungeon in my killing boots and Kabuki makeup—splitting the goddamn atom? With as much tact and restraint as I could muster, I explained that dressing up funny and witnessing acts of autoeroticism was kinda like my job description. If even a moron could see that, I inquired politely, why couldn't he?

I'll tell you why: because Joseph wasn't about ordering from the menu. Joseph wanted to eat right off of my plate. He was no more interested, fantasywise, in nuns and naughty schoolboys than he was in circus clowns and sideshow freaks. Unless, of course, I had let slip some personal reminiscence about my wild years beneath the Big Top; then he'd be all over that one like a three-legged man on a piano stool.

As a Close-Getter, Joseph needed to masturbate to my memories; nothing less would satisfy. I've seen the type before. Thankfully, however, I haven't met too many in the fetish world. Maybe that's because the dungeon is a place where deep-seated psychosexual wounds are considered standard conversation starters; you begin your digging a lot closer to the core.

Close-Getters don't say much; the uncomfortable silence makes you do the talking. When they do speak, it's to flatter and agree. The reinforcement and feigned interest make you open up; once they've detected that opening, these soulless spirits have a host to inhabit.

In Joseph's case, I think that appropriating my past as fantasy fodder was his way to avoid mining his own. It wouldn't surprise me if there was something lurking in his psyche so heinous you could hardly blame him for not wanting to examine it. But that's just life and it's no excuse. Nut up, be a man, and stay the hell out of my house.

What kills me is that I never saw it coming. I didn't recognize the violation and deceit until it was practically sitting on my grandma's linoleum kitchen floor with its dick in one hand and her Sunday purse in the other. But maybe I'm getting ahead of the story.

For months, Joseph's session consisted of basically nothing until the day I accidentally trotted out a scene from my own past. I did like the nuns did in the days when in-school corporal punishment was fading from vogue (hitting us was off-limits and thus humiliation enjoyed a glorious renaissance). I made him rap himself across the knuckles with a ruler. This instantly rekindled our session; from that moment on, all he wanted was to play young Master Bates to my tongue-clucking, finger-waggling Sister Sadist.

This was fine by me. Anybody who's done time in Catholic school will attest that the experience does leave its share of, shall we say, residue. Personally, I'd seen enough cruelty during my own twelve-year bid to keep all the Josephs in the Archdiocese going until Vatican IV.

But that's neither here nor there—I know how fashionable it is, among the hipster set, to bad-mouth your given faith. It's the theological equivalent of hating the small town you grew up in because you're afraid you might someday return. So suffice it to say that, like a good sound paddling, it hurt when it was happening but I'm awful glad I went. After all, it made me who I am today.

This is how it played out in Joseph's session: I'd take some sick, borderline-child-abuse event from grammar school and relay it to Joseph. He'd listen attentively and ask the right questions, appropriately horrified and titillated, eager to begin the reenactment. Before we got to playing, I'd go back and retrofit the story so that it would contain an opportunity to catch Joseph jerking off.

For example: One year, during Lent—I believe it was third grade—Sister Agnes told us how very pious children would wear a rough, tight cord around their waists from Ash Wednesday to Easter Sunday, so as to atone for the sins of the world. And though this wasn't a direct order from her to us, she did note that it had spared other children from the eternal fires of hell—and that the cord should be about one and a half inches shorter than the waistband of our uniforms. We were just learning fractions and using grown-up scissors in art class; the opportunities for extra credit seemed almost limitless, Sister Agnes hinted.

So I made Joseph don the cord, tight and itchy like a miniature hair shirt. And I knew that once bound, even a grown-up couldn't help but fiddle with it, to get some play, make it looser, decrease the discomfort. And once Joseph was down there fiddling, I knew the chronic masturbator would also go on to call the tune. Innocent enough, as far as perversions go.

But here's where Joseph, the Close-Getter, really began to reveal himself. One afternoon, I was all tapped out—not out of lurid school stories, just lacking the desire to tell one. So, in related news, I started telling him about my new apartment, and my bedroom window, which is directly across the street from a convent, and the bedroom window of a nun who used to teach at my grammar school. I told him that I couldn't blame anyone for peeping into her window any more than I could fault her for peeping into mine.

Quite by accident, I let it slip that my apartment wasn't just some random rental; I'd inherited the place from my grandmother. That sweet and tough old Sicilian lady had lived there some twenty-three years until her death a few months ago. She'd bequeathed the place to me on her deathbed, shrewdly realizing that a rent-controlled, laundry-room-on-premises pad might be just what I needed to bring some sanity, some stability to my life—and ensure that I wouldn't move away from my family anytime soon.

I loved that woman with all my heart and today I cherish even the humblest of my inherited possessions—the big spaghetti pot, her wig collection, her autographed copy of Howard Stern's *Private Parts* (I tell no lie—next to the Bible, this was the only other book she owned). These were all a part of her very last gift to me.

I admit that I may have gotten a bit lost in the reverie when I related this to Joseph. But then I snapped myself back into character and started chatting about the strange late-night habits of nuns and the things they might do within their late-night bedroom walls.

But it was too late. Joseph was done with nuns and now he wanted my grandmother. Feigning a respectful curiosity, he wanted to hear about her saint statues and Miraculous Medals, her housedresses, and her cooking utensils. He wanted to hear about the nights I'd slept over, as a young girl, when she'd bathe, manicure, and powder me, and we'd stay up late watching Mary Tyler Moore, Carol Burnett, and Cher.

He wanted to know about these sleepovers: Did I ever peep in on the nuns in the middle of the night? Did I ever masturbate while peeping? Would it be possible, seeing as we were friends and all, for him to sleep over sometime, masturbate, and peep? Finally, I'm sickened to say, he wanted to know if I thought Grandma had ever peeped out that window.

That was when I knew I had a Close-Getter on my hands. It's also when I turfed him, plain and simple. I didn't even dignify his filth with a reason or reply—that would only give him more to work with. See, you can dis my religion and piss on my church; you can hardwire all my sacraments into your Wank Databank, but there's sacred, mister, and then there's *sacred.*

You keep your filthy masturbator's mitts off my dead relatives or you'll have Granny to answer to. She always did try to warn me, in her own inimitable way: Ruby, watch out for assholes and strangers. She'd left out the part about Close-Getters, though—I guess that's because they're no different from the first two.

—

In reliving these experiences, it's easy to see what I regarded as the most unpardonable sin a client could commit: Thou mayest frolic and play dress-up, and speaketh with the falsest of tongues, but thou shalt not get personal with thy mistress.

This would explain why, in my hour of greatest duress, I decided to do unto my clients in a similar fashion. In short, I got real—and real ugly.

BIZARRO RUBY

Maybe it's the headlines, the kind you see only a certain time of year. You know, when summer's just about overstayed its welcome and only mayhem can ensue. It's the season commonly associated with Altamont, Attica, Manson, riots, Son of Sam, celebrity bitings, Woodstock '99, and so forth.

It's like the codes of civilized behavior have been suspended from July Fourth until Labor Day. Every time I can bear to look around, I see people feeling just a little too free to let it all hang out. I'm telling you, it makes me uneasy.

As above, so below, goes the scripture, and so I knew that whatever weirdness was happening in the streets would eventually be reflected in the types of requests I'd receive, the characters I'd meet in the dungeon. What I didn't expect is that ultimately I'd outfreak them all.

This all started when a client came in for a "verbal humiliation" session. Young kid of about twenty-one or twenty-two; by my estimation, he really had no business in my business, having simply not lived long enough to have accumulated the sexual cynicism, the emotional armor from which a session with me might release him. Anyway, his fantasy, as he explained it, was to lie on the cold stone floor, naked and masturbating, as I insulted him to orgasm.

I was having one of those days when I was in no mood to suffer fools, gladly or otherwise, so when he asked me how long a session he should book—half-hour or hour—it was all I could do to refrain from treating him to a preview of the insults he would soon enjoy.

"You sure we shouldn't go for the full hour?" he asked.

"Trust me, a half-hour will do just fine."

I told him to disrobe and assume the position, and I'd be back in a minute. I had nowhere to go and nothing to do; a little presession in-out is a stock mistress trick designed to heighten client anticipation. Also, it helps make that all-important separation between the reality of our civilized consultation and the fantasy that I am this merciless hell bitch come to Earth solely for the purposes of berating him to the point of ejaculation.

But somewhere between freshening my lipstick and dressing a blister, I had the weirdest little moment. You know those times when Superman becomes trapped in the Bizarro universe? Let's just say I left Dungeon #2 the regular me—well, the regular mistress me—and returned, newly Band-Aided and brooking no bullshit, as Bizarro Ruby.

It was a difference that totally cinched the session. Whereas the regular Ruby would have delivered a steady stream of standard-issue insults—*What a horny little beast, can't help but play with yourself, can you?*—bringing him home in a respectable ten, fifteen minutes, Bizarro Ruby was not content with conventional, safe, impersonal bad-mouthing. In the Bizarro dungeon, the fourth wall was about to come crashing down.

I slammed into the room and slapped a stopwatch down on the metal supply shelf. Understanding his cue, Client Boy gripped himself and began his business.

"This is ridiculous," I stated calmly. "Do you realize that you're wasting your money? I've got a blister the size of a turnip on my foot, and I just don't feel like dealing with you." I had loads more to say, except I never got the chance to say it. It appeared we had a huge hit on our hands—or rather, all over his.

It was the shortest-running show of my entire career. One minute, thirty-six seconds. As I basked in the satisfaction of a job well done, Client Boy wiped up and stepped back into his khakis. He grinned sheepishly. "Guess I'm glad I didn't pay for the full hour, right?"

I poked at my blister. "Does this look infected to you?" I asked.

This humiliation and degradation, a.k.a. "Doing the Rude," is a kind of scene that has always seemed really wrong to me. It's pretty much as it sounds; you take a man and say mean things to him, or make him do something embarrassing. The essential redundancy of this activity is perhaps best expressed by my old e-mail buddy Fred. With characteristic candor, he writes: "Why would I need to go someplace special to get put down and shit on? I get enough of that at my own job!"

True enough, and while I'm sure he's echoing the sentiments of many, Fred doesn't work where I work. I'm reminded of another thing people always say to me, about how nice it must be to have a job where I get paid to take out my aggressions and frustrations on people. *You must be so relaxed and pleasant by the time you go home.* Yeah, I'm rolling in clover, I am.

The sad truth is that they are not *my* aggressions and frustrations I am getting out on anyone. When I'm face-to-face with a client, I've got no more urge to make him hump the punishment horse and bray like a donkey than you would.

And that's what irks me about these so-called humiliation scenes: it's all rubber knives and phony bloodstains. No one's really embarrassed in a way that he has not expressly requested. It's not like you're risking the kind of bodily harm that such envelope-pushing might cause you in, say, a heavy flogging scene. Anyone who's seen the damage that a thoughtlessly placed ball-chain whip can cause would certainly agree: words, they really can't hurt you.

So if you want to talk about alternate planes and topsy-turvy universes, consider the great unwritten rule of my workplace. You know all those lowly, crawling worms, all those stinky, sniveling, fart-breathed bastards that grovel and beg and cry and wheedle at my feet? In this reality, my job is to serve *them*.

But fear not, fair citizens; Bizarro Ruby is out to change all that. Fact is, this has been my kick for the last couple of weeks—giving myself a vacation from the faux-mean, canned-mistress routine. This month, I'm the real, raw deal. When a guy comes to me and wants to be fake degraded as the hostage in an S&M sex-slave camp, forced to disrobe at whip-point, I'll gladly make him remove every stitch—toupee first.

Some stiff investment banker wants to play Mistress's Slutty Lesbo Girlfriend at the Titty Bar? Fine by me, but my girlfriends have class; they don't bump and grind like dollar-dancing whores while I stab at them with a dildo I know they can't take and they know I'll never use. My bitch does interpretive ballet, and she knows all the words to "It's a Long Way to Tipperary," even the tricky ending. And if she fucks up, well, there's always that dildo we call the Widowmaker.

And speaking of dicks, don't ask me what I think of yours. You really don't want to know. And don't ask me what I want to do at any given moment. Because while Mistress Ruby might confess that her most heartfelt desire is to make you fellate her high heel like the stiletto-blowing whore that you are, Bizarro Ruby will tell you that she wants you to leave your money and . . . leave her alone.

—

Soon after that, I left the dungeon for good. Like so many disgruntled employees, I had my own ideas as to what, exactly, would constitute a blaze of glory. I won't go into any of them here, except to say that the idea of leaving Leona something to remember me by— anything from cockroach infestation to a visit from local authorities—provided me with hours of wicked fantasy.

In the end, the drama that attended my departure was strictly internal. Even my Bizarro campaign and my Close-Getter blowout were significant only to me. And while I had no plans for when I'd leave exactly, I saw all the signs that the end was coming. This was the same way I'd quit smoking and broken up with I can't tell you how many boyfriends. Months of brooding and silent dissatisfaction; then one day, apparently out of nowhere, the ashtrays disappear, the boyfriend finds his suitcase out in the hall.

So I'm not being cute when I tell you that the moment took me by surprise. I remember exactly where I was when it happened: in Dungeon #2, doing a session with a rubber fetishist named Herb. He was a perfectly nice client, not to be blamed for any of this. He was just a paunchy, pushy, bespectacled munchkin of an estate lawyer who happened to be loving rubber when my internal clock ran out.

And he was indecisive. He couldn't decide whether or not he wanted to suck my glove or lick the hem of my latex skirt. We went back and forth for about fifteen minutes: *Well, Herb, suppose you lick my skirt first, and then, if you do a real good job, I'll let you suck the glove.*

But that wasn't good enough—turns out that Herb only liked to lick black rubber and suck the red and unfortunately, the skirt I was wearing was crimson and my gloves were gray. Lately, this kind of dickering depressed me; I'd begun to contemplate how many of these inane client preferences were robbing me of brain space that I could be putting to better use. I had a column due the next day, for instance, a fact that could only make Herb's dilemma more aggravating.

But I didn't get mad; I didn't get sad—it was far beyond that. What I got was indifferent.

I'm not even sure if I knew what I was about to do.

"I'll be right back," I said.

"Great," Herb said. "And you'll bring those latex chaps, just in case?"

"Yeah, that," I said, as I closed the door behind me.

It was a truly transcendent moment. Which is my way of saying that I don't remember much of it, so over time, I've appropriated that last scene from *An Officer and a Gentleman,* when Debra Winger is swept away from the factory amid a chorus of cheering coworkers. Except in my case, there was no Richard Gere; there wasn't even any fetish gear. I took nothing from my locker, crammed with thousands of dollars' worth of outfits and implements. And while the workers in our fantasy factory were cheering, it had nothing to do with me: Erica, in the throes of a painkiller addiction, had just OD'd on *All My Children,* and the doms were going wild. In all the commotion, no one saw me swipe a sweatshirt from the coat closet, step into my sneakers, and walk out onto the streets of midtown Manhattan.

And then the weirdest impulse overtook me. I would stop and have a drink. Toasting my freedom was not remarkable; it was my choice of bars, one of those awful prefab "Irish" sports pubs, where the derelict quotient was not high enough to allow a woman in Adidas, rubber, and Abercrombie & Fitch to sit and drink unnoticed. But it also had a big bay window from which I could observe the traffic between Lady Leona's and the number 6 train—the same one that would take Herb back to his office.

There are people who'd say I was looking for closure. I prefer to think of it as a kind of satisfaction—the giddy payoff of a juvenile prank. For instance, you might light a bag of dog turds in front of a neighbor's door, but if you're not hiding in the bushes, watching him stomp out the flames, you've only done half your job.

It didn't take that long, maybe a beer and a half, before Herb came walking by. He looked so small and puzzled, walking down the street with a limp I don't think I'd noticed before. In fact I realized I'd never actually seen him in daylight and so his appearance, even though I was expecting him, was startling—like spotting a movie star in a supermarket. I could only imagine the sequence of events that must have taken place.

First, he'd have to get impatient, step outside Dungeon #2—having clothed himself or not—interrupt the other girls and their soaps, then suffer their annoyed assurances that I was coming back. Eventually, the manager would appear, and offer to refund his money or let him see another mistress, cursing me all the while. In a couple of hours, however, annoyance would give way to concern, and even my most unfeeling coworkers would begin to wonder if I was okay.

I'm sure I should have been touched by that, but at the time, it seemed like the funniest thing I'd ever seen or done. I laughed and laughed and ordered another beer, but the bartender wouldn't let me pay for it. Suddenly, being an adult had never felt so rewarding.

—

I hung up my whip for good after that. I never did another session, at Leona's or elsewhere. I didn't miss the dungeon, and this time around, I wasn't worried about the lost income. I'd inherited a little bit of money from my grandmother—not a huge sum, but enough to give me time to contemplate my next move.

Once I'd dropped my clients and given away what was left of my wardrobe, all that remained of my mistress career was the column I wrote about it. And now, even that was coming to an end.

I knew that signing off was the right thing to do. Like so many jobs, it had started off as a tremendous opportunity, a chance to do something new. But now it was chaining me—so to speak—to a world that I was done with. There were other things I wanted to write about, and thanks to my seminotoriety, I started getting the opportunity to do just that. I shook hands with my editors, and we made plans to phase me out.

Fortunately—or maybe not—one thing I hadn't yet lost was my skewed sensibility, what I like to call the Lens of Leather. No matter where I looked, I saw everything as an exchange of power, or the playing of a role, or as a negotiation between people—for good or for bad. The dungeon just happened to be a very extreme version of how people lived every day. As above, so below—it seemed like even the Holy Bible was acquainted with the S&M underworld.

SEX FOR SANTA

Blame it on the holiday shopping season, but lately everything I do feels like a transaction. You know how it is: you send cards to people who send them to you; you give gifts in social defense. An invitation to dinner means you bring the wine; if your pocket's tight, an ornament for the tree will suffice.

It's easy enough to keep a running tally of what's given versus received. But it's practically impossible to keep track of what you do for the spirit of the season, and what you do for the sake of the scorecard.

Even the most basic human exchanges seem fraught with obligation. Just the other day, I was catching up with Desi, and I swear that what we had wasn't a conversation; it was two people taking turns talking. I bought time at the mike by listening to her business, and in turn, she listened to mine.

It was pretty much understood that you could score extra airtime if what you were saying directly concerned the other person. But when she told me that she was earning her Christmas money by selling her ass on the weekends, I stopped eyeing the meter and started paying attention.

Purely for the sake of the record, here's a little peek at the price list: hand job, $30; blow job (dry), $50; blow job (with swallow), $75. Straight sex, $125; a half-and-half (half suck, half fuck), $150. S&M play not culminating in intercourse, $200 per hour; with sex, $250. Anal sex costs a cool $300, or this darling Prada bag she's been eyeing since Fashion Week. [http://www.puckerup.com/main.htm]

All prices are accurate as of press time, but if she's got her period, tack on a 25 percent surcharge. Extras such as dirty talk, costumes, and orgasms (hers, real or faked) are either itemized or negotiated ahead of time for a generous tip.

But even if you could afford her, don't bother me for her phone number. Desi's got but a single client: Graham, her boyfriend, whom she services exclusively. They're madly in love. They've been together for years.

It's only fair to mention that Desi's a person quite unlike you and me. Stalkers, voodoo, and stints in nonspecific institutions are things that touch her life on an everyday level. She's the type of person who'll say things like "Once, when I was getting kidnapped *a lot . . .*" with complete unblinking earnestness. So if it weren't for my keen reportorial instincts, I would have tossed off the sex-for-Santa business as just another Desian phenomenon.

But then I started digging around. I asked a random sampling of friends—gay, straight, fetish, et cetera—if they'd ever exchanged sex for cash in an established romantic relationship. Everyone understood right off that we weren't talking socially sanctioned prostitution, such as marrying for money, say, or letting a date grope you in the orchestra seats he scored for *Les Miz.*

What surprised me was how many people knew the thrill of cash on the nightstand for a willing body in the bed, even when that body was one they usually slept with for free. Maybe the money that changed hands wasn't enough to threaten the nation's economy, but

I do know a kink when I see one: money, fetish of fetishes, the ultimate sex toy.

I think we can be pretty sure that wherever there's sex, there's a sex industry. And it's hard to work in a dungeon as long as I have and not regard a supervised orgasm as a perfectly reasonable purchase. Most people think that men who frequent dungeons—or any other sex business, for that matter—are seeking something they just can't get at home. But that's only part of the picture. It's a big, crazy world out there, and the truth is, many clients could probably find their session in the private sector if they really wanted to.

Whether or not they'd admit it, most of my clients come to me for the sense of going someplace special to have their needs met. In that way, it's not so different from pampering yourself with a facial or a custom-made suit. But because what they're looking for is sexual in nature, it's also about the sneaking, the seediness—and the paying for the privilege.

As a mistress, I'm well aware of how money plays in the picture. It's a liberator, and it simplifies what might otherwise be a complex exchange. You plunk down your money to get what you want— within reason, of course—and none of what you don't. By accepting that money, I've agreed to suspend my own emotional needs for the time being. Unlike a "real" relationship, you won't have to address my insecurities as to how your cross-dressing affects me, much less where this affair is going—unless, of course, that's what you *want* to talk about. Ultimately, you're not really paying me to play dress-up with you. You're paying me to disappear when you're done.

But that's no big deal in an exchange between strangers. What fascinates me is how money changes the game when there's already a deep emotional history. Certainly, there's the element of liberation—the buyer calls the tune, the player does the dance. But through that, a tremendous amount of knowledge can be gleaned.

To put it another way: I know what a lover will do for me if he knows he stands to gain something down the line. And even if he's pleasing me out of love, there's still that sense of obligation. So let's fuck politeness for a minute and get down to raw, selfish desire. Maybe I'd like to see what he'd do if he *didn't* have to think about me. It's very much like watching someone masturbate. Factor me out of the equation, and I can sit back and watch. Maybe I'll catch a glimpse of what he really likes; and maybe, just maybe, a glimpse of what he's really *like*.

Of course, you can't start throwing bills around the bedroom without acknowledging the sheer tawdriness of it all, and that's all to the good. Sex without sleaze isn't sexy, it's procreation. If you're like me, you've been long inoculated against the seedy charms of getups and gadgetry. Christ, but I've spent so many afternoons in skintight leather that by now it's about as erotic as Granny's flowered housedress.

Money, however, never fails to be filthy. It's worn, it's dangerous, it's been around the block and laid the pavement. It represents the potential for purchases both good and bad. It's got a nasty reputation, and if you're willing to trade your body for a small stack of those greasy greenbacks, that reputation just might rub off on you.

Money, being worldly, makes the world come crashing in. The game that started as a goof—*You wanna do it? Gimme twenty bucks*—takes a sudden and serious turn. The fact that you're paying for something you'd ordinarily get for free forces you to step back and consider its worth in the world, forces you to consider your mate as someone who has a sexuality that doesn't necessarily include you.

In a way, it makes you strangers; but then again, between strangers, there's very little sense of obligation. So maybe you can't exactly put a price on affection. But a sense of appreciation, of newness—sure, I just might trade my ass for that.

BE A SLUT! BE A SLUT! BE A SLUT!

In every bar in every town across this great nation, there is a woman who will dance with you, and with abandon. Her hair has got that tousled morning-after quality to it, dark of root and frosted at the tips, and if you can't picture pulling on it, just you wait a few more beers.

Her walk is loose, as if her joint sockets have been recently greased; her lipstick looks as if it wants to be on someone else's body. When she stands, it's too close. She does not so much sit as straddle. Her panties, if she has them, can often be found in a ball at the bottom of her purse, stuck to her Binaca blaster. And she's got at least one tattoo—or stretch mark, depending on age—on a part of her body that you've got every chance of unearthing before the sun rises over the parking lot.

This woman is a slut. *Trampus americanus.*

I know this woman because week in, week out, I field half a dozen requests to make men—grown men! upstanding men!—over in her image. Indeed, if worse came to worst, I could probably float my entire dungeon career on the basis of this fantasy alone. The scourge of most women, the secret darling of men, you will find that wherever people are hung up on their own sexual impulses, the cult of the slut is alive and well and giving out blow jobs in the back rooms and dungeons of Anytown, USA, the hang-up capital of the universe.

But before we go any further, let's define our terms. I'm not talking about prostitutes here—women, and men, who will suck and fuck for money—though it's true that a certain hard-core slut faction is not averse to leasing out the pussy if it means getting a warm place to sleep from time to time. But we'll get to that later. For now, suffice it to say that if your workplace is called "the track" and there are no horses around, you, my dear, are a prostitute.

My Webster's defines *slut* as 1) a slovenly, dirty woman; a slattern, 2) a woman of loose morals, 3) a prostitute. In Webster's view, the word itself is a judgment. *Slut* is a *slur.*

But I think that if we were to be totally honest with ourselves, the word *slut,* in everyday parlance, carries more than just a whiff of jealousy. A so-called nice girl is quick to deem another woman a slut if that other woman is diverting her man's sexual attention away from her. To the nice girl, the slut is playing *fast* and *loose*— two words commonly associated with sluthood, of course—with her own sexual power, something the nice girl has been taught never to do.

Secretly, however, the nice girl suspects that while the slut may or may not be winning the mating game, she's definitely beating the pants off her in the side race—because the slut is having way more fun on the trot.

But for men, I think the story is a bit more basic. While the word still contains the insult, that insult is tempered with resentment. To your average Joe, a slut is a woman who, though suspected of being sexually active, will not give *him* the time of day (see also *bitch* and *lesbian*). At least, that's the public face of it—it's not so much a word as it is an epithet, one that is spat and hissed and hurled from construction sites and muscle cars of frustrated dickheads, commonly underscored with an obscene hand gesture.

Privately, however, it is my observation that most men would like their women to behave like shameless trollops, wanton and loose. But only under the most carefully controlled conditions: that is, for him and only him. And you'd better just cut it out when he begins to fear that he won't be able to keep up with you. In this case, the private-dancer slut is about as owned by her man as the nice girl is by sexual mores and her mother. My advice to these women: put your pussy in an envelope and mail it to its new owner. Advice to these men? Don't let the beast out of the bag if you can't handle the consequences.

A different Webster's—the unabridged version, naturally—allows a fourth definition of *slut:* a bold, brazen girl. I can back that one. In my mind, there are two kinds of slut. The first is a woman who, due to a host of self-image difficulties, possible paternal neglect and abuse, the subsequent slew of shitty boyfriends, and a modicum of spite, develops a pathological need to fuck or appear to fuck as many guys as possible. Sex becomes the only way she knows how to get attention.

Stay as far away from this creature as possible. The only way you can fix things is to make *her* problem *your* problem, and never you mind the sad and desperate origins that made her this way. The sob story that caused her not to care about herself is the same one that will land your ass in a VD clinic. Or worse.

The second kind of slut, simply put, is a woman who takes her pleasure as a man does. That means to fuck as is her wont and without guilt or remorse; when the sun comes up, her body is still her own. These women wield a profound power because they are in full possession of their own sexuality.

And they do us all a great service by weeding out the weak: the man who fears her is probably not worth your time. These women are the sex warriors, the independent owner-operators who bring great honor to our gender. They always carry their own protection, and you don't necessarily have to marry them afterward—though you may find yourself wanting to.

But let's bring this back to the dungeon. By far the best thing about S&M play is that it's a means of exploring gender roles and boundaries in ways that are often not appropriate in everyday life. So never mind what I've been up to all weekend; as your mistress, I am the antislut, the woman you can never, ever have—no matter how I act, no matter what I do. And this, in turn, frees my client up to be the person he has always admired, reviled, resented, and desired from afar: the unrepentant slut.

But why is it, exactly, that so many client fantasies require treating them as wanton women? I know you smell a theory coming, and I won't disappoint. The fact is, I've rarely seen a cross-dresser who wanted me to dress him up from wig to garters to heels and then regard him as my respected equal, a Mother Teresa meets the Queen Mother. Unless, of course, the Queen Mother is secretly blowing the royal chauffeur and Mother T. is doing something that, if I mentioned it, would cause God to smite me where I sit.

But that's an easy theory when we're talking cross-dressers; indeed, the sartorial limitations of most dungeon CD closets would turn most any man into a street-hardened tart, those being the clothes we have handy. Let's look at the noncostume dramas—the bondage, discipline, corporal, or spanking sessions—in which a client wants to pretend that his sexuality has a value that he is willing to surrender to me, for free, in the name of a minute's pleasure, or attention. In short, a slut.

I think we already have our answer here. Like it or not, in this world a woman's sexuality—her pussy, to be blunt—trades for a higher price than does a man's sexuality. Somewhere along the line, it was established that women hold the sacred box; men want the sacred box. For the love of the box, women can get men to do things— like work a fifty-hour week, take us to fancy dinners, and pretend to be interested in our feelings. In much the same fucked-up vein, the perceived value of this box, and the challenge of attaining it, creates an increased sexual desire in the male of the species—a greater horniness, if you will.

So you take a man and treat him like a loose woman, and there you get the best of both worlds: a man's libido coupled with a woman's easy access to sex. But this only really works as a session if you take the chauvinistic view I've outlined above. Because, sure, the guy will go out and work that fifty-hour week for the pussy that stays at home, but then again, that pussy's got to *stay* at home. And in that view, the mind-set that keeps the box a precious commodity is the same mind-set that keeps a woman in her place.

That's why sluts are such an asset—necessity, even—to a free-thinking, egalitarian society. The true slut—that is, the sexually mercenary woman—trades her pussy for whatever price she desires, and leaves the backroom morality brokers to sit on their hands in frustration. In doing so, she throws a real monkey wrench into the marketplace and says a big fat fuck-you to the evil forces that allow it to exist.

If that's the case, all women should be sluts. But first we've got to reclaim the title so that it reflects the pride we feel to be honored as such. Lenny Bruce once suggested that schoolchildren say *nigger* fifty times after reciting the Pledge of Allegiance. This, he felt, was the only way to destigmatize someone else's ugly epithet. We sluts would do well to follow his example.

Postscript: Life After Ruby

At this point, I've spent much more time writing about S&M than I actually spent practicing it. Working as a mistress—the ultimate contracted labor—taught me how to deal with the financial uncertainties of freelance life, and so my transition from the dungeon to the desktop was fairly smooth.

Ironically, it was Barkley the Smart Dog who rescued me yet again, with a series of appearances that paid my rent as I expanded my journalistic empire. Eventually, I started earning more money as a writer than as an inspirational canine. Until that happy day came, however, I was plagued by a single thought: Would I ever make a buck *not* wearing a costume?

In my first year after leaving the dungeon, I was obsessed with the notion of *going straight*. Mind you, I wasn't quite sure what that meant, nor did I ever come close to committing to the nine-to-five. But just as every generation must rebel against the one that came before, I think my mission was all about living life from the other side. Or at least, seeing if I was still welcome there.

I did not want to associate with colorful characters; I didn't want to hear about anybody's sex life. Most of all, I did not want to *be* a colorful character, obliged to sing my S&M standards at social gatherings, like a boozy, middle-aged Judy Garland belting out "Over the Rainbow."

Finally, thirteen months out of the dungeon, I got my wish. It was at *New York Press*'s annual party, a raucous affair held in the ballroom of the Puck Building, a venue only slightly smaller than a football field. Some old friends of mine from Austin, Texas, were in town that week, friends who'd seen me through all phases of my writer, dominatrix, writer-dominatrix, writer career.

These dear and wonderful people were very excited at the prospect of seeing their old friend as a known figure—a *personality,* if you will—at a big New York publishing party. My own feelings about this were mixed. By the time we were dressed and ready, however, I'd worked myself up to it. It's the rare individual who really and truly wants to see his friend succeed, I told myself, and it would be downright selfish of me not to deliver. I would do the dance, I would arch the eyebrow—I would be Mistress Ruby for one more night.

And then . . . nothing. Zip. Zero. Goose eggs. I should mention that the one thing this Mistress Ruby didn't do was wear her fetish gear. As it turns out, I didn't need to: No fewer than eight other women—plus one drag queen—had decked out in the latest mistress fashions and were studding the Puck Ballroom with their ominous, outrageous presence.

Meanwhile, I was recognized by no one. In fact, the only people who approached me were people I already knew, plus one cartoonist I owed fifteen bucks to and a noogie (don't ask). Oh, and a waiter who stepped forward to tell me that I had a big splotch of salsa on my jacket.

I felt bad for my friends, who in turn felt bad for me. In a last-ditch attempt to salvage my reputation as a big-city somebody, I suggested that we stop for dinner at my favorite Japanese restaurant. "Me and Hiroki (the sushi chef) are like *this,*" I offered, twining two fingers together. My friends, meanwhile, grumbled and joked on my behalf, calling those ballroom doms "poseurs" and "empty suits."

Empty suits with an attitude problem, I later found out. In the days that followed, I received a handful of impassioned e-mails—some outraged, some disappointed—about my behavior at the *Press* party. At first, I didn't know what to make of it, but as I dealt with the static, the picture became clear. Turns out that not all of the women were merely *dressed* as dominatrices; a couple of them had actually been *pretending* to *be* me.

One of these chippies had merely dubbed herself Mistress Ruby—making no claims either way—and low-browed her way through the evening, picking arguments, baring her tits, and dumping a beer on one of my favorite e-mail buddies, Fred, just as he was trying to introduce himself to "me."

First of all, Fred, I e-mailed, *Mistress Ruby does not drink beer. I drink beer, but Mistress Ruby would never be caught in public with such an uncouth beverage. . . .*

I went on to express my regret over his unfortunate encounter, and we were friends—well, friendly correspondents—once again. But I'd somehow hit on a larger point: Me and Mistress Ruby had truly and finally separated from each other. I was not, as I'd once thought, Chang to her Eng; I was Shari Lewis, and she was Lamb Chop. If I could go to a party and watch other women masquerade as Mistress Ruby, then the experience really had come full circle. Mistress Ruby wasn't my identity; she was merely my invention—an empty, if expensive, suit.

None of this is to suggest that I regret my time in leather. But I will admit that the more years I put between myself and the dungeon, the more I appreciate the experience. For one thing, I've completely dropped the notion of wanting to *go straight.*

I realize now what a ridiculous premise that is. I mean, straight like who? Straight like the artists whose work I admire? Straight like my grandmother, who hopped the wall of a Sicilian convent to come to America with no one and nothing? Straight like bankers and lawyers and doctors and politicians, the kind who used to visit my dungeon every Tuesday?

That's the central truth that I took from mistressing—that everyone's life is at least 30 percent weirder than it appears on the surface. I find that to be a very comforting, even liberating, lesson—well worth the time I spent learning it. I took other things with me as well, like the ability to apply false eyelashes and run six city blocks in pointy shoes with very high heels (though I hope I never have to). And I absolutely cannot look at a person without wondering what his (or her) deep, dark, sexual deal might be.

Nowadays, I walk around the city like one of those angels in *Wings of Desire.* My fellow citizens—freaks and weirdos, absolutely, every last one of them—speak their secret desires in a language only I can intuit. I'm afraid I'm not at liberty to disclose the nature of these revelations, but I assure you, they are all totally twisted, eminently bizarre—and gloriously human.

Acknowledgments

Dear Friends, Faithful Supporters, Literary Godfathers—as Mistress Ruby might say, *You know what you did.* . . .

D. Keith Mano, David Black, Jeff Calman, Wolff Bachner, Mary Lou Bednarski, Adam Bernstein, Will Blythe, Sister Beverly Cardino, O.P., Bruce Fizzell, Paul Good, Scott Jones, Lewis Lapham, *New York Press,* Lee H. Smith, my agent, Lydia Wills, and my editor, Jonathan Karp.

And of course, as always, my family.

Web Resources Directory

Websites in Mistress Ruby Ties It Together
   Access Place Frank Sinatra resource page
      [http://www.accessplace.com/sinatra.htm]
   Ann Rose's Ultimate Birth Control Links Page
      [http://www.gynpages.com/ultimate]
   Bondage Techniques by Dr. Bondage
      [http://www.bondageu.com/campus/drbondage]
   Grrl Wide Web Directory
      [http://www.no-men-allowed.com/directory/grrl-web/Girly]
   Hoboken Slide Show
      [http://www.hobokeni.com/slideshow.html]
   InThe80s.com
      [http://www.inthe80s.com]
   Puckerup.com
      [http://www.puckerup.com/main.htm]
   Toys in Babeland
      [http://www.babeland.com]

Some of Robin Shamburg's Favorite Websites
   Dr. Ducky DooLittle: The Site of Sexual Curiosities
      [http://www.drducky.com]
   King of All Media.com: Home of the Original Howard Stern Superfan
      Site
      [http://www.koam.com]
   The *London Evening Standard* Crossword Puzzle Page
      [http://www.thisislondon.co.uk/dynamic/lifestyle/crossword/
         top_direct.html]

Nerve.com
[http://www.nerve.com]
The Onion
[http://www.theonion.com]
Weird N.J. travel guide
[http://www.weirdnj.com]

About the Author

After a twelve-year internment in Catholic school, ROBIN SHAMBURG studied journalism at the School of Visual Arts in New York City. In 1995, she picked up the professional whip—on a dare—and ended up staying for almost two years, moonlighting as a dominatrix to supplement her freelance career. These essays are based on the *New York Press* column "Mistress Ruby's Whipping Post." A novelist, journalist, and screenwriter, she has written for such publications as *GQ, Mademoiselle, Penthouse Online, Gallery,* and *Yahoo! Internet Life.* She lives in Hoboken, New Jersey, with her Chihuahua, Carlos, and is working on her next book.

AtRandom.com books are original publications that make their first public appearance in the world as e-books, followed by a trade paperback edition. AtRandom.com books are timely and topical. They exploit new technologies, such as hyperlinks, multimedia enhancements, and sophisticated search functions. Most of all, they are consumer-powered, providing readers with choices about their reading experience.

AtRandom.com books are aimed at highly defined communities of motivated readers who want immediate access to substantive and artful writing on the various subjects that fascinate them.

Our list features literary journalism; fiction; investigative reporting; cultural criticism; short biographies of entertainers, athletes, moguls, and thinkers; examinations of technology and society; and practical advice. Whether written in a spirit of play or rigorous critique, these books possess a vitality and daring that new ways of publishing can aptly serve.

For information about AtRandom.com Books and to sign up for our e-newsletters, visit www.atrandom.com.